Geriatrics Handbook

Practical Applications for Health-Care Professionals and Patients

FIRST EDITION -UPDATED

Venkit S. Iyer, MD, FACS
David Bernstein, MD, FACP

Publisher
DYNAMIC LEARNING
Tampa, Fl

ISBN 978-1-7344701-5-4 (paperback)
ISBN 978-1-7344701-6-1 (digital)

Printed in the United States of America

DEDICATION

We dedicate this book to our parents, spouses,
children, patients, mentors and teachers.

ACKNOWLEDGMENTS

We owe a debt of gratitude to our friends and
families for providing encouragement and support throughout
our careers and through completing this book.

We are grateful to Dynamic Learning for their expertise
and assistance with editing and formatting this second edition.

CONTENTS

Preface

People are living longer. Life expectancy has doubled in the last two hundred years. We expect the number of centenarians to be over 200,000 in the next ten years. Those living into their eighties and nineties will be common. Over the next ten years, it is possible that 30 percent of the population will be retired seniors above the age of sixty-five.

Increasing longevity and aging has its positives and negatives. It is desirable to see that people are living longer, but they also face an increasing number of healthcare and socioeconomic issues. It is a well-established fact that health-care costs increase toward the end of life.

Geriatrics is a medical specialty of providing health care for the older adult. It addresses the needs of older adults. Their health-care needs differ from those of the younger population. This handbook addresses various medical problems as it relates to older patients. Prevention of health hazards and expression of compassionate care deserve as much attention as providing proper medical care. Hence, the book is divided into those sections.

Family physicians and internal medical doctors provide most of the current geriatric care in the world. Awareness of aging adults' needs, palliative care, and end-of-life issues with their emotional, moral, and financial aspects are often ignored or forgotten in the busy life of a medical practitioner. Today, medical science focuses more on short-term fixes and immediate problem-solving instead of treating the whole person, long-term wellness, or preventive care. Hence, a considerable amount of a senior's care falls on the shoulders of nurses, aides, and on family members.

The practice of geriatric medicine is not attractive to young physicians. Currently, modern technology, procedures, and frontiers of medical advances are much more attractive, exciting, and more lucrative, although geriatrics is a well-recognized field in Western medicine. The importance of geriatric care is gathering momentum in the rest of the world as more people are aging.

The authors hope this handbook will illuminate the healthcare needs of our aging.

Section 1

INTRODUCTION

Chapter 1

Importance of Geriatric Medicine and the Process of Aging

In 1909, while he was working at the Mount Sinai Hospital clinic in New York, Dr. Ignatz Leo Nascher first proposed the term Geriatric medicine to describe health care of the older adult. Since then, Geriatrics has grown into a specialty of its own, with physicians undergoing fellowship training after completing medical school and three years of training in Internal medicine or Family practice. This underscores the importance and need for special attention to the health care needs of the older adult. Since the term "elder adult" is vague, most would prefer the term "Older" adults. Geriatrics is health care for older adults, while Gerontology is the study of aging, including biological, sociological and psychological changes. The two systems go hand in hand to enable one to understand the needs of our aging population.

Aging can be chronological, stating the actual number of years one has lived or it can be biological, reflecting the state of health that equates one to comparable. A young person can be physiologically older because of medical problems, obesity, unhealthy addictive habits (substance use, excess tobacco or Alcohol, overeating, gambling) or poor lifestyle. On the other hand, an older individual can feel and look younger if they do not have these issues. We all want to live well, feel well, and enjoy an excellent quality of life until the very end.

Aging is a process and not a disease. It refers to the inevitable decline of various organ systems because of dysfunction of the DNA. Reduced functional capacity of each organ makes it difficult to withstand illnesses, injuries and insults to the body. Diseases make an aged person more vulnerable than a younger person. Vice versa, diseases are not to be mistaken for aging. Older people may have multiple dysfunctions and disabilities; they may be on multiple medications. In addition, they can be more susceptible to internal damage, such as intracranial bleeding from a minor trauma or a fracture of femur from a slip and fall.

The major reason for aging is genetics, and we have little control over it. Observe the skin and subcutaneous tissue of a five-year-old and that of a seventy-year-old. The face of the five-year-old is chubby, full and shiny. Make a pinch- it fills back instantly. It is hard to find a vein in the arm or leg. The seventy-year-old has loose skin, with wrinkles settling in, and bags form under the chin or under the eyes. Take a pinch of the skin- you see that it is so loose, and it takes longer to return to normalcy. It is easy to find veins in the wrist, forearms and legs. What happened in the intervening time periods? The skin loses its collagen and elastin in the subcutaneous tissue during the aging process. This is just one manifestation of aging.

Human cells wear out and die because of cumulative wear and tear. We speculate that energy molecules called ATP become depleted. Another consideration is that oxygen molecules allow "free radicals" to form, which disrupts the electronic equilibrium. Telomeres that are the DNA pattern in the chromosomes shorten and break off, which leads to the death of the cell. It may be because of a built-in code that stops the cells from regenerating.

Aging may result from two factors: nature and nurture. Nature is the genetic influence and nurture is the environmental influence. Scientists believe humans beings are genetically programmed to age and die. Individual cells in the body have different life spans. Hundreds of thousands of our cells die daily, but we reproduce them as well. Stomach cells last about two days, red blood cells last 120 days, bone cells last for thirty years and so forth. Despite the reformation of cells, the body is programmed to slow down and become weak. Different living species have different life spans built into their genetic code. Houseflies live for thirty-five days, while a sequoia tree lives for 2500 years. Humans live for one hundred years.

A second cause of aging has to do with Nurture: our own making, the consequence of our lifestyle and outlook. These items are detailed in the later sections of this handbook. These are items that one can control, unlike the natural aging process. With attention to these details, along with progress in science and medicine, we have already doubled the life expectancy of human beings over the past two hundred years. It is quite possible that humans will live for 120 years routinely in the next two hundred years' time; eighty-year-old and ninety-year-old may not be old then.

Life expectancy has been steadily increasing in the world. The longest life expectancy is in Japan, eighty-four. Twenty-eight percent of the Japanese are over sixty-five. In 1900, only 4 percent of the world population was above age sixty-five. Currently, 20 percent of the population is over sixty-five, and in the next ten years 30 percent of the population could be above sixty-five. Ten thousand people are turning sixty-five every day in the USA. Women live five years longer than men, because of genetic, environmental and sociological and psychological reasons.

At the time of retirement, many individuals are at a loss. Having worked long hours and being engaged, sudden emptiness and lack of activity can be troublesome. It is reported that the Japanese couple have more friction, divorce and suicide after retirement. But there is life after retirement, and it can be enjoyable too. One needs to plan activities to fill the day and to stay engaged in worldly affairs.

To keep a certain level of self-respect, it is important for older adults to remain financially stable, connected to others, and maintain their health and independence for as long as possible. As one gets older, they become wiser, softer and more tolerant compared to their own younger age. They often become more spiritual and cherish family and friends. Maintaining good health is certainly more of a priority than being wealthy.

Adults are looking forward to "Healthy Aging" and not just aging. Healthy aging involves (1) Low number of illnesses and disabilities (2) High cognitive and physical functioning, and (3) Active engagement with life. Examples are activities such as traveling, independent living, driving, participation in sports or group activities, managing financial affairs, and enjoying cultural activities. Such activities might include fine arts, theater, sporting events, bird watching, photography and other pursuits.

In summary, aging is a natural process, and it is unstoppable since time moves in only one direction. It is a question of how long one can remain in good health and be independent and not a question of how many years one lives.

Chapter 2

History and Physical Examination of the Older Patient

History:

Taking a history and performing a physical examination should be the same for all patients. However, there are components that require special attention when dealing with the older adult.

For example, older patients are likely to have multiple medical problems and a single added problem may worsen already weakened organ systems. Senior adults may take multiple medications, both prescribed and over the counter. Even though they may present with only one immediate concern, it is important to review all the details, since there is a tendency to hide or ignore other issues. They may forget elements of their past medical history, and they are afraid to reveal too many issues to the doctor. Hence, a systematic full history and physical examination is important. Review of electronic medical records and conversations with a primary care physician and close family member or caretaker are helpful.

During the medical interview, besides obtaining medical information on the presenting symptoms, one would also investigate mental status, social interactions and functional status of the patient. A full review of all systems is necessary to avoid missing any present or past illnesses.

During the interview, encourage patients to wear items they use such as dentures, eyeglasses and hearing aids. When possible, patients should be interviewed alone to ascertain the potential for abuse or exploitation. Caregivers should be included in the interview process as well. Support from family and friends, documentations of advance directives or Living Will, and durable power of attorney are additionally important to get the clearest understanding of the patient.

Presenting symptoms: Type of complaint, nature of complaint, and duration. What makes it worse, relationship to diet or activities? What have they been doing about it? What are their concerns?

Pain: Ask about onset, was there a history of trauma or fall, location of pain, relationship to movements, relationship to food, acute or chronic, what makes it worse or lessen, intensity, radiation of pain, referred pain, relationship with sleep, relief with type of medications.

In older adults, fractures of ribs can occur from vigorous coughing, chest pain can be due to myocardial infarction or pleurisy, back pain can be due to a ruptured aortic aneurysm or compression fracture of vertebrae or metastatic cancer. Knee pain can be due to osteoarthritis, hip pain can be due to an impacted fracture of neck of femur, headache can be brain tumor, neck ache can be subarachnoid hemorrhage and abdominal pain can be due to cancers.

Medications: Inquire about all prescription drugs, dosages, frequency, prescribing doctor's name, pharmacy name and allergies. It is often preferable that patients bring the actual medication bottles. In addition, the interviewer asks about over-the-counter medications taken without prescription, dietary supplements and herbal medications. The patient may also take Ayurvedic, homeopathic or other such alternative therapy medications or concoctions.

Substance use Disorders: Tobacco, and opioid drugs are three key items of concern. How much do they indulge, how long they have been dependent, to what extent have these substances been affecting their cardio-pulmonary, neurological and locomotor functions?

Past medical history: Older patients often forget prior interventions, surgeries, and illnesses. They may not remember the dates or other details. They may not recall test results and dates. Electronic medical records are of immense help in retrieving past information. Alternatively, patients are encouraged to keep a log of their medical history. With minimally invasive procedures, such as laparoscopic surgery, interventional cardiology procedures such as stent placement or valve replacements, there are no visible scars outside the body.

Mental Status and social problems: Older adult patients are likely to have deterioration of cognitive functions, dementia, psychological problems and neurological problems which they may conceal. Sexual dysfunctions may exist but not acknowledged. Psycho-social problems, such as exploitation or manipulation, may exist with caregivers or family members. Out of fear of reprisal, this information is often repressed. Unsafe or unhealthy living conditions are also unreported. Financial issues may lead to neglect and inattention to health and personal needs.

Physical Examination: All patients should have a similar routine and systematic physical examination. In the older adult population, certain items will need special attention.

Observe gait, ambulation, attire, alertness, and family or friends accompanying the patient. Note ability to see, hear and verbalize as they enter the examination room. These observations will give certain instant impressions about the patient's wellbeing, socio- economic status, disabilities and impairments.

Vital signs- Pulse is checked in all four extremities, to determine vascular and cardiac status. Blood pressure measurements taken in both upper extremities and in supine and in sitting position looking for asymmetry indicative of blockages in blood flow.

Nutritional and hydration status: Inspect skin and subcutaneous tissue, tongue, conjunctiva, body habitus for starvation or obesity.

Head and Neck- Look for visual problems, cataracts, glaucoma, anemia, thyrotoxicosis, myasthenia, hearing problems, cerumen accumulation, dentures and gingival problems, carotid bruit to evaluate for carotid artery stenosis, thyroid nodules and enlarged lymph nodes.

Chest: Observe for emphysema, tuberculosis, chronic obstructive pulmonary disease and lung cancers.

Heart: Auscultate for aortic stenosis, congestive heart failure, cardiomyopathy and arrhythmias, including atrial fibrillation. Observe for the presence of a pacemaker.

Breasts: Examine for cancers and lumps in both men and women.

Abdomen: Examine for tumors, constipation, abdominal distension, ascites, aortic aneurysm, and hernia.

Rectal examination: Highly recommended looking for enlarged prostate, cancer of prostate, rectal cancers.

Genitalia: Examine for testicular cancers, hydrocele and sexually transmitted diseases in male patients; cervical cancers and vaginal pathologies in women.

Urological: Evaluate for kidney problems, urinary tract infections, incontinence, retention, and prostate problems.

Extremities: Examine for peripheral vascular disorders, venous stasis, deep vein thrombosis, and varicose veins. Examine for arthritis, joint and muscle problems.

Neurological: Evaluate mental status, dementia, Alzheimer's disease, cerebellar problems, intracranial problems, and psychological problems.

Functional status: Assess ability to be self-supportive, independent, and ambulatory. Look for evidence of domestic violence or elder abuse.

The goal of history and physical examination in the older adult includes not only arriving at a diagnosis and treatment plan but includes addressing personal and social needs.

Venkit S. Iyer, MD and David Bernstein, MD

Section 2

Symptom-Based Approach in the Older Adult

Venkit S. Iyer, MD and David Bernstein, MD

Symptom-Based Approach in the Older Adult

1. Abdominal Pain

The location, duration, and severity are important questions in evaluating patients with abdominal pain. Pain in the right upper quadrant is usually due to gallbladder disease. Pain in the right lower quadrant is usually due to appendicitis, and pain in the left lower quadrant is usually due to diverticulitis. Central abdominal pain could be due to acute pancreatitis or food poisoning. There can be variations, and the pain could be due to assorted reasons. Potential malignancies need consideration in all cases of abdominal pain in the older adult.

Long duration of the pain for months or weeks could be due to chronic conditions such as peptic ulcer disease, esophageal reflux, cancer conditions, Crohn's disease, or ulcerative colitis. Sudden onset of pain within one or two days is often due to an acute process such as acute cholecystitis, acute pancreatitis, acute appendicitis, or acute diverticulitis. Very excruciating and extremely severe pain suggests an acute serious pathology such as perforated viscus, gangrene of bowel, strangulated hernia, torsion of ovary, volvulus of gut, or other causes of peritonitis.

After complete history and physical examination, flat and upright abdominal x-ray, sonogram of abdomen, and CT scan of abdomen and chest are options. Depending upon the diagnostic consideration, further tests are to be considered. Treatment depends upon the diagnosis. Acute conditions will require fluid replacement, antibiotics, and surgery.

2. Abdominal Distension

One classically categorized causes of abdominal distension as caused by five Fs: fat, fluid, flatus, feces, and fetus. It is further categorized by causations such as obesity, ascites, gas buildup (intestinal obstruction), constipation, and pregnancy. Physical examination and history contribute to making a diagnosis. More tests such as ultrasound of the abdomen and CT scan can confirm the exact cause. During the examination, evidence of tenderness, rebound tenderness or rigidity, and peritonitis are assessed. Ascites may manifest as shifting dullness on percussion and fluctuation of fluid. Fluid in the peritoneal cavity can be due to free blood. Spontaneous bleeding into the abdominal cavity can be from ruptured ectopic pregnancy, ruptured abdominal aortic aneurysm, retroperitoneal hematoma, acute hemorrhagic pancreatitis, ruptured spleen, or ruptured liver tumor.

Obstruction of the intestines or megacolon, either acquired or congenital, can cause massive abdominal distension. Constipation can be slowly progressive and chronic or could be more acute because of obstructing cancers or other obstructive pathologies. Pregnancy is a consideration in every female of childbearing age; a pregnancy test should be routine in all such patients before ordering any radiology tests or surgical intervention. Besides the above causes, large tumors such as ovarian cancers or renal cancers, neuroendocrine tumors, and retroperitoneal sarcomas can present as abdominal distension. Marked enlargement of organs such as spleen, liver, and pancreas can cause abdominal distension.

3. Agitation

Agitation is a symptom complex that can manifest in diverse ways. The patient becomes restless, anxious, irrational, or aggressive. Agitation can be due to neurological problems, such as dementia, schizophrenia, or bipolar disorder. It can be due to fever, meningitis or encephalitis, and septic conditions. It can be due to drug reaction, alcoholism, or delirium. It can be due to inability to express problems such as pain, retention of urine, or restraints. Any acute illness can result in agitation.

Investigate to figure out the root cause and treat accordingly. Nonpharmacological intervention is the preferred first step. Medications used in treating agitation appear elsewhere in this handbook.

4. Alcohol and chemical dependency

The NIDA (National Institute on Drug Abuse) defines addiction as *"a chronic, relapsing disorder characterized by compulsive drug seeking, continued use despite harmful consequences, and long-lasting changes in the brain. It is considered both a complex brain disorder and a mental illness. Addiction is the most severe form of a full spectrum of substance use disorders, and is a medical illness caused by repeated misuse of a substance or substances,"* such as alcohol, narcotics and nicotine and uncontrollable behaviors around obtaining and using the substance. There are many factors that contribute to drug and alcohol addiction, including genetic and environmental influences, socioeconomic status, and preexisting mental health conditions.

Excessive use of alcohol can cause multiple organ disorders. Chemical dependency slowly creeps in and becomes a routine habit even without the knowledge of or recognition of the person. Older individuals are more affected and disabled. The consequences are both mental and physical. Alcohol affects the brain, liver, pancreas, heart, and immune system and increases cancer risk. It can cause Wernicke's encephalopathy, delirium tremens, and mood-affecting situations, violence, traffic accidents, sleep disorders, and sexual dysfunctions. Women can transmit the disorders to a newborn child if they were addicts during pregnancy. In older adults, it leads to cognitive disorders and early onset dementia. Genetic, environmental, or social factors may contribute to this medical illness as well.

5. Anxiety

Anxiety is excessive worry and nervousness about ordinary and inconsequential matters in day-to-day life. It leads to muscle tension, restlessness, irritability, and insomnia. It can also lead to impairment in social, occupational, and family interactions. Variations of anxiety disorders are agoraphobia, panic attacks, obsessive-compulsive disorder, social phobia, and substance abuse. Medications such as caffeine, corticosteroids, nicotine, psychotropic, sympathomimetic, and thyroid hormone can induce anxiety. Physical conditions such as cardiac arrhythmias, angina, myocardial infarction, endocrine conditions such as hyperthyroidism, hypoglycemia, pheochromocytoma, or neurological conditions such as epilepsy, Alzheimer's disease, stroke, and respiratory problems such COPD and asthma can induce anxiety. Treatment involves counseling, support, and therapy along with medications as needed. buspirone (BuSpar), benzodiazepines such as diazepam (Valium), alprazolam (Xanax), lorazepam (Ativan), oxazepam (Serax), and hypnotics such as Ambien, Sonata, and Lunesta may be helpful but must be used with caution in this population.

6. Arthritis

Patients refer to all aches and pains in bones and joints as arthritis irrespective of the underlying medical pathology. The discomfort could be a simple sprain of ligament or chronic rheumatoid arthritis or even metastatic cancer. Hence, it is important to take a full history and physical examination before ordering any investigations. History of trauma or sporting injury will be of short duration. These injuries are more common in the knees and shoulders. Autoimmune disorders are of long duration and involve fingers and toes.

Shoulder pain can be due to rotator cuff tears, tendinitis, frozen shoulder, or subacromial bursitis. These patients have diminished shoulder movement, pain on abduction, and arc movement. Treatment involves identification of the repeat provocative movement causing the pain and avoiding them, along with pain medications, followed by gentle exercises to strengthen the muscles. Uncontrolled pain or disability might require surgical consultation.

Hip pain can be due to fractures, trochanteric bursitis, or osteoarthritis. Hip fracture causes sudden onset of pain usually after a fall. There is an inability to walk or bear weight with restricted movements of the hip joint. X-ray or MRI will confirm the fracture, which could be in the femoral neck or intertrochanteric or subtrochanteric areas. Treatment is usually by surgical correction, such as insertion of intramedullary nails, hemiarthroplasty, or total hip replacement.

Knee pain can be due to tearing of the meniscus, cruciate ligaments, or osteoarthritis. Initial treatment of osteoarthritis is conservative. Total joint replacement is an option for unrelenting arthritic conditions.

Besides trauma, we can relate arthritis to a specific disease. The most common is osteoarthritis from overuse and aging. Other causes are rheumatoid arthritis, psoriatic arthritis, systemic lupus disorder, polyarteritis nodosa, polymyalgia rheumatica, temporal arteritis, gouty arthritis, or Paget's disease of bones. We often categorize back pain from spondylosis or prolapsed intervertebral discs as arthritis of the back. One should always consider the possibility of metastatic cancers to bones from organs such as prostate, breast, lungs, and thyroid that can present as bone pains or joint pain.

7. Back Pain

Most individuals experience back pain during their lifetime. Fortunately, most episodes are transient and because of musculoskeletal problems rather than vertebral problems. Lifting unusual weight or sporting injuries or sudden twists related to a fall or sleeping in a bad posture are common reasons. Physical examination will reveal an acute exacerbation of the pain with certain types of movement, such as bending or turning, with no neurological changes and no abdominal findings. History will reveal the pain is of short duration. Patients often remember a precipitating event. Treatment recommendations include rest, pain medications, and gentle back exercises. As the muscle sprain heals, the symptoms resolve within days.

More problematic are causes related to the vertebral column or spinal roots or spinal cord. These may involve prolapsed disc, spondylosis, nerve root compression, spinal cord injuries, and tumors of neurological origin, collapse of the vertebrae from osteoporosis, or metastatic cancers to vertebrae and retroperitoneal tumors. MRI of the spine is helpful in making a diagnosis. Treatment depends on the exact etiology. A small percentage of patients may require surgical intervention.

Excruciating and unrelenting back pain of short duration associated with hypotension and abdominal distension, or pain suggests a ruptured abdominal aortic aneurysm. A sonogram of the abdomen or CT scan will confirm the diagnosis. This is a surgical emergency and requires immediate intervention.

8. Bruising

Older adult patients often notice easy bruising and ecchymosis under the skin. It is more obvious on fair-skinned people and raises alarm for the onlookers. Part of the reason is aging itself. The connective tissue becomes fragile, and blood vessels rupture easily. Subcutaneous tissue fat, which protects the capillaries, gets diminished in volume. Varicose veins develop with aging, and they bleed externally or into the subcutaneous space. Minor traumas can cause hematoma and ecchymosis in the old. Frequent falls are possible in old age. Multiple venipunctures for frequent blood tests in patients with diabetes mellitus, renal failure, and anticoagulation therapy leave large ecchymotic areas.

Another cause to keep in mind is the side effects of medications, particularly anticoagulants and antiplatelet medications often prescribed to the older adult.

It is also important to consider elder abuse. Caregivers can get frustrated and annoyed because of the need for long-term care and the demand for frequent attention. The bruises on the backside of the body, genital areas, and grip areas on the upper arm or wrist are warning signs.

Medical conditions and bleeding disorders such as hemophilia, thrombocytopenia, cirrhosis of liver, splenomegaly, hemolytic anemia, collagen disorders, and autoimmune disorders also can cause spontaneous ecchymosis.

9. Body Aches and Pains

Older adults complain of aches and pains in various parts of the body regularly. It may not be specific to any organ dysfunction, but further investigation could lead to an underlying medical condition. We may relate these myalgias to muscle aches from activities, posture, or aging. The discomfort may be related to chronic arthritis, deep vein insufficiency, lymphedema, and cardiac or pulmonary problems. On a more acute basis, one should think of trauma, falls, sprain, or acute infections such as flu, viral sepsis, coronavirus infection, or fever. It could also be a psychosomatic problem. It is important to make a prompt diagnosis of correctable painful conditions such as acute abdomen, peritonitis, fractures, and ligament tears.

Estimates reveal that almost 50 percent of older adults complain of chronic pain. A portion are afraid to talk about their pain, or they are undertreated. It is necessary to perform a complete evaluation as to the etiology and severity of pain. Initially, nonpharmacological measures with local therapy, exercises, and rehabilitation, along with systemic nonopioid analgesics, are options. When necessary, low-dose opioids for short durations might be helpful.

10. Chest Pain

The most urgent concern about chest pain is heart attack or myocardial infarction. The pain is sudden in onset and is a deep, severe pressure sensation. It can radiate to the left shoulder or jaw or to the substernal region. It is usually on the left precordium, unrelenting and associated with tachycardia, sweating, and hypotension. Other cardiovascular conditions that cause chest pain besides acute myocardial infarction are pneumonia, esophageal reflux, pericarditis, aortic dissection, and unstable angina.

However, a variety of conditions can mimic a heart attack, and the pain can be unrelated to cardiac events. Acid regurgitation and esophagitis, peptic ulcer disease, cholecystitis, pleurisy, pneumonia, pulmonary embolism, musculoskeletal problems such as fractured ribs, muscle sprains, diaphragmatic irritations, anxiety syndromes and panic disorders, and costochondritis (Tietze syndrome) are such causes.

A thorough history and physical examination can help diagnose these conditions. Cardiac enzymes and serum troponin are elevated, and EKG will show ischemic changes in acute myocardial infarction. An ST elevation myocardial infarction (STEMI) responds to intervention with immediate coronary angiography and intervention with thrombolytic therapy, angioplasty, or stenting of the affected coronary arteries.

A chest x-ray will help to identify the pulmonary and chest wall problems mentioned above.

11. Chills/shivering

A common reason is bacteremia due to sepsis. The origin of infection could be the urinary tract, the hepatobiliary tract, gastrointestinal problems, indwelling catheters, or meningitis. Blood cultures will usually be positive in such cases. Other infections less common now are malaria, typhoid, typhus, and viral sepsis. High fever from any reason can result in rigors. Hypothermia and low temperature can cause shivering. Hypoglycemia, physical exertion, hypothyroidism, medication effects, anxiety, and stress are other reasons. Infections need immediate intravenous antibiotics and the removal of the source of the infection at the same time.

12. Constipation

Constipation is a common complaint of older adults. One major reason is inadequate fiber intake. Neuromuscular reflexes diminish with age, leading to fecal impaction. This further adds to constipation as the hardened fecal mass acts as an intraluminal obstructive object. Other factors contributing to constipation are slow motility, immobility, lack of visceral sensations because of aging, and dehydration. Metabolic causes include diabetes mellitus, hypothyroidism, hypercalcemia, and heavy metal intoxication. Certain drugs such as iron, calcium channel blockers, anticholinergics, narcotics, diuretics, and anti-Parkinsonian medications also can induce constipation.

Other conditions include cancers, volvulus, megacolon, strictures, and such organic causes of intestinal obstruction. A complete history and physical examination, including a rectal examination, are appropriate. An X-ray, ultrasound, or CT scanning of the abdomen may be helpful. Treatment depends on the underlying cause. It may require disimpaction and enemas. Stool softeners or laxatives, used with caution, are helpful. Increased fluid and fiber intake are to be encouraged.

13. Coughing

Coughing is one of the most common symptoms presenting to a primary-care, geriatric, or outpatient clinic. Cough is an effort by the body to expel irritants from the tracheobronchial tree. The cough could be as simple as aspirated fluid or food or infections of recent onset or more serious underlying pathology such as malignancy.

Recent onset of coughing along with fever or myalgias is a common experience related to flu, viral infections, upper respiratory infections, laryngitis, and pharyngitis or streptococcal infections or epiglottitis. There is often a coexisting acute bronchitis. Many are viral infections but can get suppurative with bacterial infections with productive sputum. Fortunately, these viral infections resolve spontaneously within a few days. However, in an older adult, these simple upper respiratory infections can transition into pneumonia and even death. Older adults have poor immunity. Their muscle strength is weak to cough out and expel the sputum, leading to occlusion of bronchial lumen and collapse of the lung. The recent pandemic of coronavirus infection presents as flu-like symptoms initially but rapidly progresses to respiratory problems and death among the older adult. Allergic rhinitis, bacterial sinusitis, pneumonia, and whooping cough (pertussis) are other causes.

Chronic cough and dyspnea can be due to chronic bronchitis, tuberculosis, bronchial asthma, COPD, bronchiectasis, and finally malignancies. Such malignancies can be from lung, trachea, and larynx or hypopharynx and may present with blood-tinged sputum. Smoking can induce coughing. Other causes are reflux esophagitis, aspirations, eosinophilic bronchitis.

Common antitussives are benzonatate (Tessalon Perles), dextromethorphan (Robitussin DM), guaifenesin (Robitussin), codeine phosphate with guaifenesin, and hydrocodone with homatropine (Hycodan). Commercial antitussive/expectorants have antihistamines or allergy medications added to the composition. Antibiotics are a suitable option when a bacterial illness is suspected (if there is yellow productive sputum or fever). Macrolides, sulfa, doxycycline, or cephalosporins are options.

Equally important is the identification of an underlying cause of the chronic cough. Sputum cultures, x-ray of chest, CT scan of chest, and bronchoscopic examination may be necessary to find and treat these issues.

14. Delirium

Delirium is not a symptom that the patient complains of, but something recognized by medical professionals or caregivers. The patient experiences disturbed mentation, making gibberish and disoriented comments, hallucination, and confusion. Sometimes there is agitation, tremors, or violent movements. In the hospital setting, patients pull out nasogastric tubes, Foley catheter, or IV tubing and get up or fall out of bed.

Causative factors could be alcohol or prescribed or unprescribed drug withdrawals, postsurgical, postanesthetic, effects of medications, high fever, and sepsis or head injury or meningitis and encephalitis. It can also be due to metabolic disorders, dehydration, electrolyte disorders, uremia, hepatic failure, hyperglycemia, hypoglycemia, or hypoxia. Other causes include shock for any reason, severe illness of any cause, sleep deprivation, or urinary retention.

Management requires identifying the underlying cause and correcting it. Safety of the patient is necessary to prevent injury. Over the past few decades, haloperidol (Haldol) or Librium have been used to control agitation. Quetiapine or Lorazepam are other drugs used, but we must use all medications with great caution as they have undesirable side effects and can make delirium worse.

15. Depression

Patients, family members, or caregivers may complain about persistent depression. Some older adults lose interest in all activities. There is unexplained fatigue and loss of energy, insomnia, feeling of guilt or worthlessness, suicidal ideations, inability to focus or concentrate, and weight gain or weight loss. There is a lack of motivation to do daily chores, bathe, or dress and loss of interest in pleasurable activities or in social interactions. Aging and dementia are factors. Loss of loved ones, failure in work or studies, loss of wealth, and abuse can lead to depression.

Management includes nonpharmacological measures initially, especially for short-term and mild cases of depression. Problem solving, environmental adaptations, and cognitive behavioral therapy can be helpful. Pharmacological agents such as antidepressants are helpful, but long-term can be counterproductive.

16. Diarrhea

Diarrhea is loose bowel movements with a liquid stool that happens multiple times and often out of control. It can be sudden and short-lived, as happens after food poisoning or gastrointestinal infections. Pathogens such as salmonella, shigella, Giardia lamblia, Vibrio cholera, and Clostridium difficile are well-recognized infectious agents. Many events are related to contaminated food or water. Clostridium difficile colitis (pseudomembranous colitis) is secondary to the use or abuse of antibiotics.

Diarrhea can be chronic and long-standing in inflammatory bowel disease such as Crohn's disease and ulcerative colitis. Problems with digestion and absorption of fat causes steatorrhea. Diseases such as irritable bowel syndrome, mesenteric vascular insufficiency, amebic colitis, partial obstructions and chronic constipation can present as diarrhea.

Celiac disease or nontropical sprue is a chronic condition with genetic predisposition, which leads to intestinal reaction to x-gliadin fraction of gluten. They have profound fatigue, intermittent diarrhea, and anemia. They need a gluten-free diet and should also avoid milk and dairy products since they may have lactose intolerance as well.

Certain medications (besides laxatives) can cause diarrhea as a side effect. Such medications include cimetidine, PPIs, H2 blockers, erythromycin, diazepam, digoxin, colchicine, chemotherapy agents, methyldopa, and NSAIDs.

Surgical procedures can cause diarrhea. They include resection of length of small bowel leading to short gut syndrome, subtotal colectomy, vagotomy, obesity bypass procedures, and resection of terminal ileum, which leads to lack of reabsorption of bile salts.

Treatment of severe acute diarrhea includes intravenous fluids to rehydrate the patient, antibiotic therapy to counteract the infectious process, and binding agents to reduce the diarrhea. Binding agents of use are Lomotil (diphenoxylate with atropine), Kaopectate (attapulgite), Pepto-Bismol (Bismuth subsalicylate), Rifaximin (xifaxan) or Imodium (loperamide). Cholestyramine binds bile salts and reduces diarrhea in individuals who have loss of their terminal ileum either from surgery or disease. For Clostridium difficile, treatment starts with the discontinuation of offending antibiotics and initiation of vancomycin or Flagyl (metronidazole). Another option is Fidaxomicin. We base treatment for chronic diarrhea on its underlying cause along with symptomatic therapy.

17. Dizziness

Older adults are more prone to dizzy spells, blackouts (syncope), unsteady gait, and falls. Potential causes include neurological conditions, medication effects, or cardiac conditions.

Light-headedness lasting one to three minutes after standing up or sitting up suddenly from supine position is often due to orthostatic hypotension. The blood pressure drops 20mmHg on changing the posture from supine to upright. With advancing age, there can be a decrease in baroreceptors' sensitivity or Parkinson's disease, peripheral neuropathy, hypovolemia or anemia, and vertigo. Medications can also cause postural hypotension such as medications for antihypertensives, or phenothiazines, acetylcholinesterase inhibitors, tricyclic antidepressants, monoamine oxidase inhibitors, or drugs for erectile dysfunction or Parkinson's disease.

Unsteady gait and balance problems presenting as dizziness can be due to multiple sensory impairments, such as problems with vision, vestibular function, spinal proprioception, cerebellar problems, Parkinson's disease, or lower-extremity neuropathy.

Short blackouts/syncope or dizzy spells can be because of carotid artery stenosis. These events are referred to as transient ischemic attacks (TIA) and can be a warning of full stroke in the future. An evaluation for carotid artery stenosis is indicated for this condition.

Sudden head and neck movements can induce fainting spells. This can be due to reduced vertebral artery blood flow or because of cervical spondylosis. Whiplash injuries following automobile accidents with sudden deceleration can induce similar changes.

18. Dyspnea

Dyspnea is shortness of breath mostly related to lower respiratory system problems that interfere with the exchange of oxygen and carbon dioxide. One important question in history is to know if the dyspnea is acute and short duration or if it is intermittent and recurrent or if it is a chronic and long-standing problem. One would also like to assess functional impact on the patient with ability to work or walk and precipitating factors. Associated symptoms of cough, fever, nasal congestion, chest pain, and edema of legs are to be considered.

Acute dyspnea can be due to pneumonia, acute coronary syndrome, aspiration, pulmonary embolism, cardiac tamponade, pneumothorax, anaphylaxis, panic attacks, or exacerbations of any chronic condition. Chronic dyspnea can be due to COPD, bronchial asthma, congestive heart failure, anemia, or interstitial lung disease or chronic and end-stage medical problems.

Most common causes are congestive heart failure and bronchial asthma. Other pulmonary causes include pneumonia of bacterial or viral origin, consolidation of lobes, pleural effusion, bronchiectasis, tuberculosis, sarcoidosis, fungal infections, pulmonary embolism, and COPD (chronic obstructive pulmonary disease).

Acute infections such as community-acquired pneumonia and viral infections such as flu are associated with high fever, chills, coughing with tachypnea, anorexia, and rhonchi and rales on auscultation. Chest x-ray may show areas of pneumonitis or consolidation.

In congestive heart failure, an exam reveals jugular venous distension, tachycardia, along with moist crepitus and rales on auscultation. A chest x-ray shows fluffy opacities in scattered fashion.

In bronchial asthma, there is the distinctive expiratory wheezing with withdrawal of chest wall muscles and abdominal muscles to increase oxygenation.

In COPD, there is evidence of emphysema, chronic bronchitis, and cor pulmonale with barrel chest, wheezing, and pulmonary hypertension. Chest x-ray shows transparent lung space, increased bronchial markings, hyperinflated lung, and increased heart size.

In pulmonary embolism, there is a potential for shock, hypotension, and chest pain, and it is of sudden onset, often following immobilization or surgery.

Treatment is directed toward the underlying cause of dyspnea. This may involve use of antibiotics, antihistamines, bronchodilators, oxygen, and systemic or cardiac support.

19. Dysphagia

Difficulty in swallowing in the older adult can be due to diseases or obstructive pathology or due to neurological deficits. While obtaining a history, it is helpful to inquire about the duration of the problem, associated illness, and consequences of the symptom. Dysphagia could be related to issues in the oral cavity, pharynx, mid esophagus, lower esophagus, or in the stomach. Dysphagia for solids suggests obstructive pathology, while dysphagia for liquids and solids suggests neuromuscular pathology.

Oropharyngeal dysphagia refers to problems of solids or liquids moving from oral cavity to upper esophagus. Patients typically gag, cough, or aspirate as they start swallowing. Problems with dentures, gingivitis, or oral cavity lesions can interfere with eating and can be present as difficulty in swallowing. Aging by itself can slow this process, resulting in 10 percent of older adults having episodes of silent aspirations.

Carcinoma of the esophagus is a serious condition and often presents with weight loss. Carcinoma can also be in the fundus or cardia of the stomach or at the GE junction. Upper GI endoscopy with biopsy is an intervention to confirm the diagnosis.

Esophagitis can be due to acid reflux or hiatal hernia or Plummer-Vinson syndrome. Barrett's esophagus has columnar cells in the lower esophagus, which can lead to carcinoma of the esophagus. Stricture of the esophagus can occur following ingestion of caustic materials and poisoning. Pill-induced esophagitis can also lead to painful swallowing and dysphagia.

Neurological problems affecting swallowing include stroke, achalasia cardia, pharyngeal muscular dysfunction leading to pharyngeal diverticulum, scleroderma, Parkinson's disease, Alzheimer's disease, multiple sclerosis, upper motor neuron disease, and injury to glossopharyngeal or laryngeal nerves following surgical procedures in head and neck region. Swallowing studies and speech studies are components of a full neurological assessment. If recurrent aspiration is discovered, placement of a tube feeding via gastrostomy or jejunostomy is a way of avoiding recurrence.

20. Dyspepsia

Dyspepsia is chronic recurrent pain or discomfort in the epigastric or upper abdominal region. Patients complain of indigestion, nausea, acidity, and loss of appetite. These symptoms might be due to any upper GI tract problems such as peptic ulcer disease, hiatal hernia with reflux esophagitis, gastritis, alcohol abuse, use of aspirin or NSAIDs, carcinoma of the upper GI tract, or motility disorders of esophagus.

A complete history and physical examination followed by targeted testing is appropriate. An upper GI endoscopy and ultrasound of the abdomen are part of the initial round of testing. A CT scan of abdomen further delineates correctable pathology.

One would direct treatment toward the underlying cause, such as medications for peptic ulcer disease. Often patients self-medicate with antacids or Pepto-Bismol before seeking a medical evaluation.

21. Dysuria

Dysuria is defined as difficult or painful urination. It commonly affects older men due to prostate problems. In this condition, patients also complain of hesitancy, frequency, incomplete evacuation, and incontinence. Painful micturition can be due to urinary tract infections, which are more common in women. Escherichia coli is the predominant organism in over 50 percent of cases. Other common bacteria include Proteus mirabilis, Klebsiella, Serratia, and Pseudomonas aeruginosa.

Urinary tract infections are caused by conditions such as enlarged prostate (benign or malignant), stones in the bladder or kidneys, decrease in bacteriostatic prostate secretion with aging, increased vaginal pH, decreased lactobacillus, anatomic weakening of pelvic floor, diabetes mellitus, cerebrovascular accidents, neurological disorders including Alzheimer's disease, and fecal incontinence causing retrograde contamination. Besides dysuria, patients also complain of fever, chills, frequency, hematuria, suprapubic abdominal pain, functional incontinence, and nausea. Urine tends to be foul smelling, and urinalysis and urine culture provide confirmation.

Prevention of urinary tract infections requires judicious use of indwelling urinary catheters. In acute situations such as the postoperative phase, recommendations include removal of catheters as soon as possible. Attention to nutrition, hydration, and behavioral modification can be helpful. In chronic situations, it is better to have a long-term indwelling catheter rather than frequent instrumentations. Suprapubic catheters are a convenient approach and less likely to provoke severe urinary tract infections.

It is unnecessary to treat asymptomatic bacteriuria with antibiotics. Therapy of documented urinary infection requires antibiotics such as amoxicillin, cephalexin, and sulfa such as TMP/SMZ (trimethoprim/sulfamethoxazole). Quinolones were used in the past but because of the side effects and development of resistant bacteria, they are reserved for resistant urinary tract infections based on urine culture results.

22. Excessive Bleeding Tendency

Patients notice easy bruising and black-and-blue discoloration even with minimal trauma, venipuncture, or compressive grips. Minor cuts bleed for prolonged time. Patients present with spontaneous internal hemorrhaging into the retroperitoneum or into GI tract. Lethal situations can arise with intracranial bleeding. Older adults are more susceptible to bleeding complications from falls or due to comorbidities such as renal failure, liver failure, malnutrition, malignancies, amyloid disease, vascular disorders, and various medication effects.

Easy bruising and bleeding can be due to side effects of certain medications, such as anticoagulants or antiplatelet agents. Some medications' effects can be reversed, but others do not have effective antidotes.

Excessive bleeding can also be due to underlying diseases that affect the coagulation system in the body, such as cirrhosis of the liver or idiopathic thrombocytopenia or hemophilia. Diseases of arteries and veins can make them susceptible to rupture. Examples are aneurysms, arterial wall weakness, and varicose veins.

The aging process can lead to easy bleeding due to loss of the integrity of connective tissue and the immune system. Elder abuse and domestic violence can initially present as bruising in unusual locations.

It is important to identify the cause and take corrective steps. Laboratory testing of coagulation profile, bleeding time, and liver chemistries are appropriate. Dosages of medications may need refinement. New medications to correct coagulation abnormalities can be initiated.

23. Fainting

Fainting episodes or syncopal attacks are more common among the older adults than a younger cohort. From these brief episodes, patients may recover spontaneously, or the event may suggest a more significant underlying medical process. The presenting symptom of syncope could be a fall.

The fainting or syncopal event could be due to transient ischemic attacks (TIA), where ministroke symptoms appear related to carotid artery stenosis from atherosclerotic plaque formation or an arrhythmia. The plaque materials can break off, or clot materials can form and go downstream as micro emboli into a cerebral artery. Left alone, it could be a forewarning sign of a full stroke in the future. Other features of TIA can be transient blindness of either eye, temporary weakness of one side of the body or one extremity or slurring of speech. These patients need carotid duplex scan as an initial test to be followed by MR angiogram or CT angiogram. Carotid endarterectomy would be a consideration in cases of severe carotid artery stenosis.

Another cause could be cardiac. Atrial fibrillation has gained greater recognition as a cause for TIA. Asystole or severe bradycardia and vasovagal syndromes can cause fainting spells. Heart blocks from conduction disorders can induce lengthy periods of asystole. Drugs, such as digoxin, can induce severe bradycardia. EKG, Holter monitoring, and echocardiogram will help to identify cardiac pathology.

Postural hypotension can cause fainting spells such as when the person changes position from supine to sitting. Medication side effects are another culprit. Opioid drugs, antihistamines, alcohol, sedatives, and antipsychotics can cause fainting spells.

Neurological disorders of any nature can present as syncope. Cerebellar lesions and intracranial diseases can cause similar episodes. Hypoglycemia and hypocalcemia can induce syncope. Psychological causes need to be considered. Hypovolemia, dehydration, heatstroke, and hypotension can precipitate fainting. Postprandial hypotension can present as syncope.

Once the underlying cause for fainting/syncope is determined, treatment is selected accordingly.

24. Falls

Older adults fall more often than their younger counterparts. Falls are harbingers of further problems that can deteriorate into their eventual demise. Falls and fainting spells often occur in tandem. The same factors that cause fainting can cause a fall. In addition, frail older adults often have unsteady gait, balancing problems, visual and hearing impairments, and musculoskeletal weaknesses. The various medications prescribed or taken over the counter can cause unsteady gait as well. Such falls could easily result in fracture of long bones or cause dislocation of major joints. Medical professionals should investigate patients who complain of frequent falls for all the causes of syncope. These individuals need protection in their homes with safety measures such as grab bars in bathrooms. Most visits to the emergency room trauma unit are from falls rather than true life-threatening injuries.

25. Fatigue

Fatigue is a common symptom experienced by older adults. Fatigue does not have a specific organ-related issue, but patients say that they just feel weak and lack energy. In a younger population, we can relate fatigue to overwork or stress. In the older population, it can result from a serious underlying medical condition. Every patient complaining of fatigue needs a thorough evaluation.

Any organ failures such as cardiac failure, renal failure, chronic infections, pulmonary problems, endocrine issues, hepatic insufficiency, gastrointestinal problems, malnutrition, anemia, and cancer conditions can zap their energy. The list of medications with the side effects of fatigue is lengthy. Mental depression and psychological disorders can reduce motivation. Chronic fatigue is a syndrome by itself. Treatment requires non-pharmacological measures to provide support, help, and motivation as well as pharmacological measures to alleviate pain, insomnia, depression, and underlying medical problems.

26. Fever

Fever is a symptom that the patient often notices, or it is a measurement of elevated body temperature performed in a health care setting. It is up to the physician to find the cause of fever, while also providing symptomatic treatment to reduce the body temperature.

Most commonly, fever is because of an infection, bacterial or viral. The usual culprits are urinary tract infection or respiratory tract infections. However, fever can occur from other clinical situations such as viral sepsis as in dengue fever, chikungunya, HIV infections, influenza, coronavirus or viral pneumonia, or parasitic infection such as malaria, amebiasis, or hepatobiliary infections such as cholecystitis, or cholangitis. It can also occur in the setting of infected intravenous lines, phlebitis, infected indwelling implants such as Infusaport and pacemaker, or bacterial endocarditis or infected vascular grafts for renal dialysis or necrotizing soft tissue infections, diabetic ulcers, decubitus ulcers, or peritonitis from perforated appendicitis, diverticulitis; or it can be heatstroke or even psychogenic. Postoperative fever can be due to wound infections, intra-abdominal abscesses, anastomotic leaks, and atelectasis of lungs, aspiration pneumonia, or infected implants. Heatstroke is from exposure to environmental heat. When the cause of fever is not clear, the condition is classified as fever of unknown origin (FUO). In recent years, we have discovered most FUO are due to connective tissue diseases.

Systematic history and physical examination will lead to clues in diagnosis. Other investigations will include blood count and routine chemistries, cultures of blood and urine or sputum, and x-ray of chest. Further tests may include sonogram, CT scan, or MRI.

It is helpful to bring the body temperature down using tepid sponge, cool blankets, and antipyretic medications such as aspirin or acetaminophen. More important is to treat infections with appropriate antibiotics, find, and remove the source of infection. This may involve surgery such as appendectomy, drainage of abscesses, debridement of infected tissues, bowel resections, and removal of infected catheters or intravenous lines. As the infectious process resolves, fever also subsides.

Daily temperature monitoring in graphic forms is a useful tool for following the progress of these patients.

27. Forgetfulness

Forgetfulness is common in our fast-moving society. With aging, it increases in severity and frequency. However, significant forgetfulness is a symptom of neurological disorders such as Alzheimer's disease, dementia, stroke and head injuries, substance use disorders including alcohol abuse.

Alzheimer's disease is characterized by memory loss with difficulty in recalling basic information, names of friends and family members, places, or past events. In addition, there is language and learning impairment and a deterioration in executive function. The diagnosis can be elusive because patients are often in denial, and close family members consider the insidious onset as part of aging.

Amnesia is the sudden total loss of memory, which is usually due to head injuries or acute encephalitis or meningitis or brain tumors, either primary or metastatic.

Patients with cognitive decline need help from family members or caregivers. Programs that help with activities of daily living (ADLs) and attention to nutrition, physical activities, and diet are helpful.

28. Gangrene

Gangrene is the death of macroscopic areas of tissues or body parts. Most commonly they are because of loss of blood supply to that part of the body. Less commonly they are due to infections, trauma, frostbite, or autoimmune disorders.

The gangrenous part becomes black with no sensation, no bleeding, and no movement. Ischemia causes the area to become shriveled and nonviable. Patients may describe preexisting symptoms such as intermittent claudication or rest pain in the calf muscles. Minor trauma such as nail cutting or a minor infection leads to further rapid deterioration, and the area can become gangrenous.

Gangrene can be dry or wet. Dry gangrene occurs when the ischemia is slowly progressive, allowing the area to shrivel. Medical professionals note occlusion of the arterial tree in one or more locations on vascular studies such as an angiogram. Wet gangrene occurs when there is a suppurative, acute, necrotizing infection such as in diabetic foot or when the arterial and venous occlusions are sudden and massive. The limb becomes blue, cyanotic, pulseless, edematous, and gangrenous. Gangrene can occur in the gastrointestinal tract because of conditions such as superior mesenteric artery occlusion, volvulus, adhesions, strangulated hernia, and internal herniation as well as from severe acute infections such as acute gangrenous cholecystitis.

A workup includes identification of the cause of gangrene and taking corrective steps. Intraabdominal conditions require emergency surgery and resection of the obviously gangrenous parts. In the lower extremities, intervention is necessary, such as stenting or vascular bypass and amputation of the gangrenous tissue.

29. Geriatric obesity

There is a tendency for older adults to become obese. This is often due to a lack of activities, both physical and mental. Excess consumption of carbohydrates, adult-onset diabetes mellitus, fluid accumulation from congestive heart failure, renal failure, and liver cirrhosis further contribute to weight gain. Metabolic syndrome occurs where muscle mass diminishes and abdominal fat increases with age. Depression, dementia, and emotional problems can lead to habits of overeating.

30. Hallucinations

Hallucinations are imaginary occurrences that a patient experiences, which could be visual, as seeing things, or auditory, as hearing things, or mental imaginations. Sometimes it is a sensation of crawling insects or smelling odors that are not present. It is more common in older adults and psychologically challenged patients. Causes can be multiple, such as dementia, medication side effects, use or dependence on substances such as cocaine, LSD, marijuana, amphetamine, or heroin, or alcohol intoxication. Other considerations include neuropsychiatric disorders such as schizophrenia, bipolar disorder, stress, postanesthetic or postsurgical status, trauma, high-altitude or decompression syndrome, brain tumors, meningitis and encephalitis, epilepsy of any type, high fever, severe infections, admission to intensive care unit, isolation, severe illnesses from any reason, multiple organ failures, uremia, hepatic failure, and electrolyte imbalances.

The brain is challenged or deranged to cause these hallucinations. They can make the patient react in such a way that it can cause harm to themselves or to others, or it can lead to agitation, aggression, anxiety, and insomnia. The medical professional will need to diagnose the underlying cause and take corrective action. In the meantime, symptomatic treatment with medications to reduce anxiety, depression, and violence might be necessary. Caregivers assume the role of helping to protect the patient from harming themselves or harming others.

31. Headache

Headaches are common. Most headaches are transient and resolve with the passage of time. They are usually due to stress, vision problems, common cold or influenza, or sinus infections. Treatment includes analgesics such as aspirin or Tylenol (paracetamol) and rest.

The physician must investigate severe and constant headaches. Headaches could be due to a subarachnoid hemorrhage, impending rupture of intracranial aneurysms, brain tumor, metastatic cancers, arachnoiditis, encephalitis, meningitis, severe viral sepsis, or migraine headaches. Psychiatric and psychosomatic conditions can present as headaches in unpredictable forms. Uncontrolled hypertension can cause headaches. Certain medications such as nitrates, calcium channel blockers, and histamine blockers can cause headaches as well.

One may associate headaches with nausea, vomiting, or vertigo. A cluster headache is episodic and felt in the supraorbital, orbital, and temporal and vertex areas. The etiology is not clear, could be genetic. Migraine headaches present in the temporal region. The associated visual disturbances can precede the onset with blind spots and squiggly transparent lines in the visual fields, both of which are related to spasm of the retinal arteries. There is throbbing pain associated with an aura, vomiting, and dryness.

One associates nuchal or occipital headache with subarachnoid hemorrhage. Temporal arteritis can cause headaches in the temporal region.

Physical or mental stress may cause musculoskeletal or tension headaches. They are associated with neck spasms, muscle tenderness, and cervical spine problems.

When in doubt about the cause of the headache, a CT scan or MRI of the brain is most appropriate. Symptomatic therapy for pain control is by analgesics. Physicians recommend bed rest and correction of underlying pathology.

32. Hearing Problems

Hearing deteriorates as a normal part of aging. One estimates that 70 percent of those over eighty years of age have hearing impairment. It affects communication ability and can cause accidents, injuries, and isolation.

Sometimes the hearing loss is due to simple accumulation of wax (cerumen) in the ear canal. Eardrops that soften the wax followed by irrigation of the ear canal are quite effective. More hardened wax material may have to be removed by a specialist in ear surgery using instrumentation. Other causes of conduction defects include foreign bodies, tumors, perforated eardrum, chronic otitis media and chronic sinusitis with Eustachian tube dysfunction.

Most hearing deficits are because of sensorineural hearing loss because of inner ear disease. Causes leading to this can be due to age (presbycusis), noise damage, infections such as viral, bacterial, or fungal labyrinthitis, meningitis, cochlear damage, Lyme disease, herpes zoster, autoimmune inner ear disease, vascular disorders or systemic diseases causing cochlear damage, ototoxic medications, acoustic neuroma, Meniere's disease, trauma, or radiation therapy to head and neck region.

Investigations include audiogram, tuning fork test, conduction studies and audiological examination.

Treatment involves correcting the problem when possible. The patient may need assistive listening devices or hearing aids. A variety of hearing aids are available. One now recognizes that long-standing hearing deficits are another contributor to cognitive decline and dementia.

Cochlear implants are a choice for patients whose underlying condition includes loss of cochlear function.

33. Heartburn

Heartburn is a common symptom experienced and is more frequent in older adults. The most common cause is reflux esophagitis, secondary to hiatal hernia and GERD. Acid and food contents reflux into the esophagus, causing irritation and inflammation of this area. Part of the reason is that the lower esophageal sphincter has slid to supra diaphragmatic position, making it incompetent. Other conditions that can mimic heartburn include acute myocardial infarction, acute cholecystitis, esophageal motility disorders, and peptic ulcer disease.

Spicy food, postprandial state, obesity, and supine position aggravate the symptoms of heartburn. The regurgitated gastric contents can get aspirated, resulting in laryngitis and coughing spells, sleep apnea, or aspiration pneumonia. Acid reflux can also lead to chronic anemia, upper GI bleeding, and esophagitis and stricture formation. Esophageal malignancy can occur because of Barrett's esophagus, where the lower esophageal mucosa transitions to columnar epithelium.

The workup would include twenty-four-hour pH monitoring of the lower esophagus, esophageal manometry, upper GI endoscopy, and barium swallow.

Treatment includes dietary modifications, use of antacids, H2 blockers, and proton pump inhibitors. A later option would include surgical correction, usually laparoscopic Nissen fundoplication or modifications thereof.

34. Hematemesis

Vomiting of blood is a frightening event and could be a life-threatening problem. Patients usually go to the emergency room in panic. Vomiting of blood must be differentiated from epistaxis, where the patient may be just spitting blood along with bleeding from nostrils.

Cirrhosis of liver with portal hypertension causes esophageal varices and gastric varices. They can rupture and cause massive hematemesis. Other causes of hematemesis are gastric ulcer and duodenal ulcer, Mallory-Weiss tear of distal esophagus, severe esophagitis, erosive gastritis, Dieulafoy's lesions of the stomach, GIST (leiomyoma) of stomach, carcinoma of stomach, irritation caused by indwelling nasogastric tube, instrumentations, post-upper-endoscopic procedures or post-surgical procedures, retrograde jejunogastric intussusception, and aortoduodenal fistula.

Patients required rapid evaluation with a thorough history and physical examination and prompt arrangements for upper endoscopy, which can be diagnostic as well as therapeutic. Aggressive fluid resuscitation and transfusion of blood are initiated to address potential hypotension and shock. Depending upon the exact diagnosis, therapeutic interventions with either endoscopic methods by open surgical methods or by interventional radiology are options to be considered.

35. Hiccups

Hiccups are spasms of the diaphragm, making the patient develop sudden spurts of laryngeal noise with closure of the vocal cords and uncontrolled inspiration related to the diaphragmatic contraction. Hiccups commonly occur during hurried swallowing of food bolus. Taking water or liquids relieves it.

Other causes are subphrenic abscess, esophageal reflux disease, peptic ulcer disease, and tumors of head and neck or chest cavity, malposition of pacemaker leads, viral sepsis, and postsurgical changes. Drinking carbonated beverages, temperature changes, emotional stress, and alcohol intake are other reasons. Infections such as meningitis, encephalitis, irritation of vagus nerve, or phrenic nerve for any reason—stroke, head injury, electrolyte imbalance, medication effects, post anesthesia, hepatic failure, renal failure—are contributing factors. Sometimes no obvious reason is found, and the patient will experience disabling hiccups for several days.

It is important to find the cause of hiccups and take corrective steps. Simple remedies such as breath holding or Valsalva maneuver, breathing into a paper bag, drinking ice water, or eating small meals are options. Xylocaine jelly orally and antacids are options in the treatment. Medications such as baclofen, chlorpromazine, and metoclopramide are added options. Surgery to inject and block or disrupt the phrenic nerve to ease the diaphragmatic contraction is the option of last resort. Emotional support an appropriate therapy as well.

36. Incontinence of Stool

Incontinence of stool is yet another embarrassing symptom that the patient is hesitant to share. It affects older adults, especially as they age and become incapacitated.

Weakness of the pelvic floor and anal sphincter mechanism contributes to this. Another reason would be trauma and postsurgical or postpartum complications. Colon resections, small bowel resection with short gut syndrome, gastric bypasses, and radical pelvic surgery can lead to incontinence of stool. Conditions that cause loose stool or diarrhea cause frequent bowel movements. Neurological disorders, spinal cord disorders, radiation therapy, and chemotherapy side effects are contributing factors. Fecal impaction and constipation, acquired megacolon, immobility, lack of activity, and medication side effects are also factors. Loss of sphincter tone may be evident in patients with prolapse of rectum, prior same-gender sexual activities, and frequent instrumentations or trauma or following complicated pregnancy. Dementia, including Alzheimer's disease, schizophrenia, and psychological disorders, can reduce proper bowel functions.

Treatment involves finding underlying pathology and corrective steps. Binding agents such as cholestyramine or Kaopectate are a choice. Antidiarrheal agents such as Lomotil and Imodium can help reduce diarrhea. Attention to perineal hygiene and prevention of decubitus ulcers and perianal excoriations are essential to avoid unwanted complications. Application of topical zinc oxide and use of disposable diapers are helpful. Cholestyramine would help those who have short gut syndrome or who had resection of terminal ileum. Regular bowel habits, bulk diet, and encouraging the individual to use toilets at regular intervals and perineal exercises are of value. Surgical repair of damaged sphincter mechanism is a choice in suitable cases. A colostomy with care of the bag may be better than having to lie constantly in stool and resultant perineal ulcers for selected bedridden patients with colonic problems.

37. Incontinence of Urine

Urinary incontinence is one of the embarrassing symptoms facing older adults, and they try to hide it for as long as possible. They consider it as a stigma rather than a medical problem that causes emotional, psychological, and social distress. It is more common among women due to pelvic floor weakness following pregnancy and childbirth. Left untreated, the problem deteriorates with age, leading to depression, sleep disorders, and recurrent urinary tract infections.

There are three types of urinary incontinences—urgency incontinence, stress incontinence, and overflow incontinence. In the urgency incontinence, there is an overactive bladder when the bladder contracts spontaneously, leading to a sudden urge to void even if the bladder is not full. This problem is common among men with prostate problems, such as BPH (benign prostatic hypertrophy). In stress incontinence, the pelvic muscles and sphincter are weak around the urethra, allowing the urine to escape with minimal stress. This could happen following sneezing, laughing, coughing, lifting, exercise, falls, or any type of reason when the abdominal pressure suddenly increases. This problem is more common among women. A constant drip of urine is a third type, where there is an overflow that happens following hypertrophy of the prostate, radiation therapy, or surgery in the pelvis.

One estimates that 40 percent of the population above the age of fifty have urinary incontinence. Factors such as diabetes mellitus, obesity, high blood pressure, and urinary tract infections can affect the urinary bladder function. Pelvic floor exercises, known as Kegel exercises, can strengthen the muscles that control the bladder. Training techniques such as holding micturition until reaching a bathroom can help. Reducing unnecessary fluid intake can help while traveling. Surgery is possible in severe cases that do not respond to conservative measures.

38. Jaundice

Jaundice is yellowish discoloration of conjunctiva, mucous membranes, and skin secondary to elevated levels of bilirubin in the blood. In the newborn, it may be a normal process of neonatal physiological jaundice, or in childhood, it may be due to congenital anomalies or hematological anomalies.

In the older adult population, jaundice is usually due to liver disease or biliary obstruction. Liver disease can be from advanced cirrhosis of liver from excessive alcohol abuse or from chronic congestive heart failure resulting in cardiac cirrhosis. Hepatitis A, B, or C can occur related to viral infection or contaminated food. Obstructive jaundice is usually because of stones in the gallbladder, stones in the common bile duct, or carcinoma of the head of the pancreas compressing the distal common bile duct or, even more rarely, carcinoma of the bile duct.

Liver chemistry reveals elevated bilirubin levels. Elevated levels of conjugated bilirubin suggest obstructive jaundice, and elevated levels of nonconjugated bilirubin suggest liver parenchymal disease. Transaminase liver enzymes are highly elevated in hepatitis. We often see alkaline phosphatase elevation in obstructive jaundice.

Physical examination revealing a painless, steadily progressive jaundice with a palpable gallbladder (Courvoisier's gallbladder) and clay-colored stool suggests carcinoma of head of pancreas. Fever and chills suggest cholangitis, likely due to common bile duct stones. Subacute onset of jaundice in a younger patient associated with mild fever and nausea is probably viral hepatitis.

A workup would include a sonogram of the gallbladder and common bile duct followed by CT scan or MRCP. An ERCP may be indicated based on the patient's progress; it would serve both diagnostic and therapeutic purposes in cases of common bile duct stones.

Treatment depends upon the diagnosis. Stone diseases and cancers usually need surgical intervention. The treatment of hepatitis is both supportive and based on the identity of the viral agent. New therapies have been effective.

39. Loneliness

Loneliness is a significant problem facing society, and older adults are not immune. Loneliness and isolation can cause depression and anxiety. There is a difference between loneliness and isolation.

Isolation or being alone is when an individual is physically separated from other humans, while loneliness is when the individual feels alone even in the company of others. Loneliness can be due to aging and loss, such as a spouse or friends. Other family members and children may be busy with their own activities and work. At times, the older adult may be bedridden and in a nursing home with few visitors. Lack of mobility, inability to drive, and functional incapacity leave the individual home bound and further isolated.

There is no easy medical or social solution. The isolated older adult often relies on family and friends as caregivers.

Individuals need to make personal efforts to stay connected with other people by taking part in group activities. Reading daily newspapers, watching television, and making phone calls are ways to reduce boredom. Extreme cases may need medications to combat depression and anxiety.

40. Lump in the Breast

We must consider a lump in the breast of an older adult as cancer until proven otherwise, while fibroadenomas and fibrocystic disease are common conditions found in a younger population.

The duration of the lump—associated pain or ulceration of skin, nipple discharge, family history of cancers, prior ovarian or uterine cancers, and menopausal status—are relevant in the history. Careful palpation of the lump as to its size, mobility within the breast tissue, and tethering to the skin is necessary. Examination of axillary and supraclavicular lymph nodes for any enlargement is necessary.

Mammography may reveal a spiculated mass or associated microcalcification. A core needle biopsy is a suitable next step using ultrasound- or mammogram-guided technique.

Based on biopsy results, further management can start. Surgery, radiation therapy, hormone therapy, and chemotherapy are modalities of treatment in options. Choices of surgery are wide, local excision or lumpectomy, simple mastectomy, or modified radical mastectomy for curable cancers. In addition, the status of the lymph nodes in the axilla is assessed with sentinel node biopsy. If the sentinel node is positive for metastasis, then a complete regional axillary node dissection is an appropriate option. In patients with limited life expectancy and poor quality of life, one can do either just a lumpectomy or a simple mastectomy for local, regional control with no further treatments.

For others, adjuvant therapy is a choice after the surgical phase of treatment is completed. Treatment options are based on staging of the disease, presence or absence of regional metastasis or distant metastasis, hormone assay results, and pathology of the tumor. If the tumor is large or if it has spread to regional nodes or if it is insensitive to hormone therapy, then chemotherapy is recommended. With an early diagnosis and treatment, a better cure rate is expected.

41. Lump Under the Skin

It is common for patients to present with a palpable mass under the skin. Masses may be recent in onset while others may be long-standing. A careful history and physical examination will guide the diagnosis and treatment.

A soft, semi fluctuant, painless mass with slipping edges that has been present for a long time is probably a lipoma and multiple masses is common. These lesions can be excised under local anesthesia.

A sebaceous cyst appears as a very subcutaneous mass with a punctum attached to the skin, with clear margins, sometimes infected. They can be excised with an elliptical incision of the skin around the punctum.

Enlarged lymph nodes can suddenly appear as masses under the skin. It appears as a spherical, deep-seated but subcutaneous mass with slight mobility and with clear margins and firm consistency. They appear mostly in areas of lymph nodes such as the neck, axilla, groin, and epitrochlear region. Most are infectious in nature, but malignancy, either primary lymphoma or metastatic from another primary cancer, must be considered. Diagnostic options include either a fine needle aspiration for cytology or an open excision biopsy of one of the lymph nodes.

Primary lymphomas can be Hodgkin's disease, lymphosarcoma, or leukemia. Metastatic malignancy can arise from the breast, thyroid, visceral organs, lungs, skin, or hidden areas in the head and neck. Thoroughly search for the primary and treat accordingly.

Most enlarged lymph nodes are from processes. They can be bacterial, viral, or spirochetes. Cat scratch disease, HIV infections, other skin infections, and viral sepsis are examples.

A soft, well-defined, painless mass around the wrist joint is usually a ganglion cyst. It is the accumulation of synovial fluid related to a tendon or joint. Complete excision in the operating room is a choice if they are symptomatic.

Other subcutaneous masses are neurofibromas, metastatic deposits, or rarely histiocytomas. Excision biopsy of them will confirm the diagnosis.

42. Malnutrition in older persons

Older adults are prone to malnutrition for a variety of reasons. They may have poor dentition, a lack of appetite, chronic illnesses, medication side effects, neglect and abuse, mental disorders, gastrointestinal disorders, and dehydration. Weight loss and vitamin deficiencies can also occur. Special attention will be needed to keep their nutritional status with balanced amounts of fluids, proteins, and supplements.

43. Pain in the Legs

Older adults often complain of difficulty in functioning due to what they describe as "My leg hurts." It may be due to knee pain or ankle pain related to arthritis, or it could be calf muscle pain related to arterial ischemia or related to deep vein thrombosis or pain in leg because of neuropathic conditions. Hence, it is important to do a complete history and physical examination and pinpoint the area of pain and cause.

Intermittent claudication is arterial ischemia of calf muscles. With aging, there is plaque build-up inside the arteries due to atherosclerosis. Patient complaints of pain in the calf muscles when walking or exercising. Resting relieves the pain. The ankle-brachial index, which is normally 1, is reduced, suggesting obstruction to the arterial blood flow. As the ischemia worsens, the claudication distance reduces, and eventually rest pain develops. A further workup includes duplex ultrasound or MR angiogram or contrast angiogram. Surgical or endovascular intervention are options to correct the obstruction.

With deep vein thrombosis (DVT), there is a sudden onset of pain in the calf muscles. The pain can be elicited by palpation of the calf muscles or tenderness while dorsiflexion of the ankle. Lack of ambulation is a contributing factor. This can happen when one is bedridden as in postoperative phase or following major illnesses. It can also happen during long flights or car journeys when one is sitting in the same position for extended periods. Ultrasound of the calf veins and deep venous system is confirmatory of the clots. Anticoagulants are prescribed intending to prevent pulmonary embolism.

Orthopedic problems such as osteoarthritis, traumatic muscle and bone injuries, and other types of arthritic syndromes can present as pain in the lower extremity made worse on any type of movements.

44. Panic Attacks

Psychosomatic problems happen in the older adult population. Panic attacks can mimic serious medical problems such as heart attacks, respiratory problems, or cerebrovascular accidents. The underlying reason could be depression, dementia, schizophrenia, or bipolar disorder.

Patients can manifest symptoms of tachycardia, hyperventilation, tremulousness, flushing, sweating, anxiety, insomnia, choking sensation, chest pain, nausea, abdominal pain, unsteadiness, and light-headedness.

These symptoms are an extreme anxiety disorder. It can be posttraumatic stress disorder, obsessive-compulsive disorder, or simple anxiety disorders. Certain medications such as caffeine, nicotine, and psychotropic drugs can induce anxiety. Withdrawal of psychoactive substances associated with dependency such as alcohol, cocaine, heroin, sedatives, and benzodiazepines can also induce anxiety.

Management requires both nonpharmacological support (cognitive behavioral therapy—CBT) medications to control anxiety and addressing the substance use disorder.

45. Pressure sores

Pressure sores, also known as decubitus ulcers, are a genuine problem for those who are bedridden and non-ambulatory. Usually, they occur on the coccygeal area, trochanteric areas, and heels, which are the areas in constant contact with the bed. Initially they appear as reddish patches and later lead to subcutaneous tissue necrosis and fluctuations. Eventually, the overlying skin breaks down, leaving open ulcers, which get infected very quickly. Tissue necrosis can be deep and wide, and the infection can have a systemic impact. It is important to prevent decubitus ulcer formation by turning the body often, ambulating, using a pressure relieving or a water mattress, and using pads over these areas. In assessing these patients, issues in consideration are the patient's mobility, activity level, nutritional status, and immune status. Once the decubitus ulcer is detected, immediate wound care precautions are provided. This may include wide debridement of devitalized tissues, the use of antibiotics based on tissue culture and sensitivity, and the application of local dressings.

46. Rashes

Skin rashes can occur abruptly or long-standing. The recent onset of skin rashes is usually due to an allergic reaction. It could be something the person encountered, such as poison ivy or insect bite, scabies, or it may be a reaction to medication or food. Most rashes resolve spontaneously. Those who continue to spread or get worse will need antiallergy medication such as antihistamine or corticosteroids.

Contact dermatitis and morbilliform drug eruptions, herpes zoster eruptions, and actinic keratosis are other entities.

Long-standing skin rashes can be due to psoriasis, scleroderma, purpuric rashes, rosacea, autoimmune disorders, collagen disorders, cirrhosis liver, vascular ectasias, or seborrheic dermatitis. One will have to differentiate them from skin cancers such as squamous cell cancer or amelanotic melanomas and congenital birthmarks, stasis dermatitis, and verruca vulgaris.

47. Rectal Bleeding

Patients will notice blood in the stool when it is obvious, such in the commode or on toilet tissue. They may not notice slow GI bleeding or slow upper GI bleeding that can present as dark stool or melena. This form of rectal bleeding is detected by doing an occult blood test of the stool. Red blood in the stool causes alarm and sometimes panic. Examining the patient will lead to a diagnosis.

Hemorrhoidal bleeding is common among adults. Hemorrhoids are engorged veins bulging under the rectal mucosa. They can burst and bleed. This type of bleeding is painless, bright red, splattering the toilet, associated with bowel movement, and unmixed with stool. A rectal examination will show blood on the examining finger, but a proctoscopic examination will show that the stool in the rectal ampulla is brown, thus confirming that the bleeding is coming from the anal margin. Hemorrhoids treatments include rubber band ligation or sclerotherapy or by doing hemorrhoidectomy.

More grave concern in the older population is carcinoma of rectum. The diagnosis is often delayed as the patients defer a medical evaluation assuming the rectal bleeding is caused by hemorrhoids. The bleeding is slow, often mixed with the stool, and burgundy colored. Rectal examination can reveal a palpable irregular tumor mass in the rectum. A biopsy will confirm the diagnosis. Treatment will require surgery, such as abdominoperineal resection, followed by radiation or chemotherapy if appropriate.

Another frequent problem in older adults is diverticular disease. The usual source is the sigmoid colon, but it can arise from anywhere in the colon. The bleeding is profuse and is maroon colored and mixed with stool. Most of these episodes stop spontaneously. Patients will need a full colonoscopic examination to recognize the general area of a source of bleeding. Persistent bleeding may require surgical resection of the involved segment of colon.

Other causes of bleeding are fissure in ano (fissure in the anus), rectal trauma, angiodysplasia of colon, and massive upper GI bleeding presenting as rectal bleeding because of the rapid transit.

48. Rectal Pain

Pain in the anal or perianal region can be very disconcerting and can become an emergency. Acute pain in the anal region is usually due to one of the following three reasons: fissure in ano, perianal abscess, and thrombosed external hemorrhoid.

Fissure in ano is a tear in the anal mucosa, and since it is in the ectodermal part of the anal canal, it causes pain from the somatic nervous system's innervation. The tear can be caused by a hard stool, constipation, or idiopathic. Pain is felt during defecation. There may be a line of blood along one side of the stool, and the fissure may transition to a chronic fissure. In the acute phase conservative therapy using xylocaine jelly, stool softeners and sitz bath are recommended. Nitroglycerin ointment and Botox injections are also tried. Once the fissure becomes chronic, surgical intervention with a fissurectomy and/or sphincterotomy are considered.

Perianal abscess is an acute, suppurative, severe infection in the anal or perianal region secondary to a crypt abscess that expands to the soft tissues. There is associated fever, bulging, and discomfort and tenderness, but it may not have fluctuation. A needle aspiration will reveal pus. A Pelvic sonogram or CT scan can be performed but is often unnecessary. The abscess needs to be widely drained in the operating room. Efforts are made to identify a fistula in ano that may be a contributory cause. Patients are placed on broad-spectrum antibiotics.

External thrombotic hemorrhoid appears suddenly as a painful cherry-like bulge at the anal margin. It is due to rupture of a subcutaneous vein under the loose anal skin. In the initial stage, it can be enucleated under local anesthesia and blood clot removed. Once it becomes solidified, enucleation of the blood clot will be difficult. Then it is better to excise the entire thrombosed hemorrhoid under local anesthesia.

49. Restlessness

Restlessness is a symptom of agitation, anxiety disorder, or psychosis. It could just be a personality disorder, or it could be because of underlying medical problems, such as thyrotoxicosis, uremia, toxicity, drug reactions, electrolyte imbalance, or neurological diseases.

Restless leg syndrome is a separate entity where there are involuntary movements of one or both legs at nighttime or bedtime, resulting in insomnia. Dopamine agonists such as pramipexole or ropinirole are suggested for treatment. Carbidopa-levodopa is another option for treatment.

Anxiety is normal when facing uncertainties, tests, and events of importance or adventures. However, when it exceeds the normal threshold to cause breakdowns or disruption, then it becomes an emotional problem.

50. Sexual Dysfunction

Older adults, both male and female, face sexual dysfunctions as they advance in age. A combination of physiological changes, psychological factors, and lifestyle issues causes it. Medical problems, diseases, and medications create further dysfunctions.

In the male, erectile dysfunction or ED is a most common and personal problem. With advancing age, testosterone levels fall, the urge for sex reduces, and erections become soft and short, and hypogonadism occurs. Diseases such as diabetes mellitus, neurological disorders of all types, spinal cord problems, vascular disorders of all types, and prostate and bladder problems further aggravate the dysfunction. Medications for treatment of enlarged prostate such as finasteride or dutasteride cause erectile dysfunctions. Various other medications, chemotherapy for cancers, radiation therapy, and postsurgical complications, particularly following pelvic surgery or radical prostatectomy, are other reasons. Smoking, alcoholism, hyperlipidemia, hypertension, and Parkinson's disease are contributory factors.

Medications of phosphodiesterase type 5 inhibitors such as Viagra, Stendra, Levitra, or Cialis are effective in improving function.

Alternatives such as vacuum-assisted devices, intraurethral suppositories, and intracavernosal injection of vasodilators are effective but less desirable than taking an oral medication. Surgical procedures such as penile implant or other steps are considered but less often since the advent of phosphodiesterase type 5 inhibitors.

In the female, multiple conditions such as dryness of vagina, dyspareunia, prolapse of uterus, cancers of uterus or ovary, and fall in estrogen levels, fall in testosterone levels, cystitis, vaginal infections, and Bartholin cyst contribute to sexual dysfunction. Emotional, psychological, or marital problems can add to the mix. Medication side effects, cancer treatments, and radiation therapy are further contributors to female sexual dysfunction. Counseling, testosterone patch, estrogen cream, and estradiol tablets or rings may help women.

51. Skin Lesions

Skin lesions become more common as individuals age. With exposure to sun and wind or certain medical conditions, different skin lesions appear. Most skin lesions are benign, but health professionals must inspect skin thoroughly to detect the less frequent but serious malignant lesions.

The three common malignant skin lesions are basal cell carcinoma, squamous cell carcinoma, and malignant melanoma. Exposure to the sun is a factor contributing to each.

Basal cell carcinomas have a dark or pearly color with rolled edges, can ulcerate, and can rarely spread to lymph nodes, but it is the least malignant of the three. The patient complains of a lesion that breaks down periodically and bleeds and does not heal. Treatment is local excision. Mohs surgery is often recommended since basal cell carcinomas occur commonly in the head and neck region. Squamous cell carcinoma has no pigmentation, appears as raised or slightly ulcerated skin lesions, sometimes with scaly appearance, with distinct margins, and can spread to regional nodes. They need wide radical excision. Melanoma, usually pigmented, appears as a mole or papule with itching sensation and ill-defined margins and can spread to regional lymph nodes and to distal organs by bloodstream metastasis. Since melanomas are the most aggressive type of cancers, they need wide-margin clear excision and regional lymph node dissection.

Benign skin lesions include seborrheic keratosis, acne, sebaceous cysts, skin warts, and actinic keratosis.

Other skin lesions are related to an underlying medical condition, such as psoriasis, rosacea, and bullous pemphigoid.

52. Sleeplessness

Insomnia is a widespread problem for older adults. They have difficulty in initiating sleep, maintaining sleep, and have inferior quality sleep resulting in daytime fatigue, irritability, mood disturbances, and daytime sleepiness.

The cause of insomnia could be psychological disorders, neurological disorders, or medical problems. Stress, daytime sleeping, and certain medications can cause insomnia. Other agents that cause insomnia are furosemide, beta-blockers, pseudoephedrine, theophylline, caffeine, antidepressant medications, corticosteroids, cimetidine, nicotine, and alcohol. Sleep apnea is the repetitive cessation of breathing during sleep, which in turn wakes up the person intermittently. Restless leg syndrome can interfere with falling asleep.

Measures that can improve sleep are setting regular sleep hours and waking time, avoiding daytime sleeping, avoiding strenuous exercise or a large meal before sleeping, avoiding caffeine, nicotine, tea, alcohol before sleep, and ensuring a comfortable sleeping environment with minimal noise, light, and temperature.

Medications that can help in inducing sleep are temazepam (Restoril), zolpidem (Ambien), zaleplon (Sonata), eszopiclone (Lunesta) and low-dose doxepin (Silenor). These medications can increase the risk for falls, contribute to cognitive decline, and dependency.

53. Swollen Legs

Patients often notice edema of their legs and bring it to the doctor's attention. Their legs feel heavy and uncomfortable, and they can elicit the pitting nature of it. However, there are other conditions where the edema is nonpitting and feels hardened.

It is important to perform a complete history and physical examination. The duration of the edema, any precipitating causes, associated symptoms of cardiac or respiratory disorders, whether the edema is unilateral or bilateral, whether it is pitting or nonpitting, are useful data.

Unilateral edema of leg is due to a local cause, and bilateral edema is due to a systemic cause.

Sudden onset relates to acute infections, venous thrombosis, or lymphatic obstruction, and they are usually unilateral edema. Sudden onset in bilateral edema can be due to congestive heart failure, renal failure, or nutritional deficiency.

Long-standing nonpitting edema on one side is usually due to lymphedema. This can be primary or secondary. Primary lymphedema is congenital lymphedema precox. Secondary lymphedema can be because of filariasis, where the lymphatics are occluded by the filarial worms. It can also be due to chronic venous stasis and chronic venous insufficiency when the subcutaneous tissue becomes hardened and indurated due to long-standing venous back pressure.

Recent onset of unilateral edema can be due to deep vein thrombosis. There is associated calf vein tenderness and a positive Homan's sign. Confirmation is with a sonogram of calf veins. Treatment depends upon the exact etiology. Fluid restriction, diuretics and correction of underlying systemic disorder are useful. Deep vein thrombosis requires anticoagulation. Patients are advised to avoid sitting in the same position during long journeys.

54. Swelling in the Groin

Patients may notice swelling in the groin, or the physician may detect it during routine examination. Common items to consider are hernias, either inguinal hernia or femoral hernia, or enlarged lymph nodes in the groin.

Hernia is a protrusion of abdominal contents through a defect in the abdominal wall. With inguinal hernias, abdominal contents can protrude through the deep inguinal ring into the inguinal canal and into the inguinal region or even into the scrotum. With femoral hernias, the protrusion is through the femoral canal.

The inguinal hernia can be congenital or acquired. It can be a direct or indirect inguinal hernia. A direct inguinal hernia is due to weakness of the floor of the inguinal canal. The hernia presents as a straight bulge, and often it may have bladder, bowel, or preperitoneal tissue behind it. They may not have a true sac. Hence, it is better to push the direct hernia inward and just repair the floor. By comparison, an indirect hernia has a sac, which is the peritoneal lining, and it enters through the deep inguinal ring, traverses the inguinal canal, and comes out through the external ring to present as a bulging in the groin or into the scrotum.

Hence, an indirect hernia needs isolation of the sac and high ligation of sac along with repair of the floor of the inguinal canal. Most hernia repairs involve placement of a mesh in the floor to strengthen the abdominal wall.

Scrotal swelling can be due to hydrocele or hematocele. They need to be differentiated from a large inguinoscrotal hernia. Femoral hernia presents as a globular mass just below the pubic tuberosity and medial to the femoral artery pulsation.

Enlarged lymph nodes in the groin can be confused with a femoral hernia. Usually, the lymph nodes are multiple, bilateral, and have a spherical shape with distinct edges and slightly mobile with no expansile impulse on coughing. There may be other areas of enlarged systemic lymph nodes in such cases.

55. Tingling and Numbness

Tingling and numbness are a symptom of peripheral neuropathy. Patients may experience this in both feet and both hands, described as glove and stocking syndrome.

Diabetes mellitus is a common underlying cause. Other causes of peripheral neuritis include lead poisoning, medication side effects, collagen disorders, renal failure, metastatic malignancy, chemotherapy, hypothyroidism, alcohol dependence, smoking, and toxins. Unilateral neuropathy can be due to nerve entrapment syndromes, nerve compressions, postsurgical changes, Guillain-Barre syndrome, spinal cord compressions, leprosy, and demyelinating processes.

Nerve conduction studies are helpful in diagnosis. It is important to warn patients to avoid even minor injuries since they may not feel pain. Classical diabetic foot abscess festers under the tissue with minimal symptoms until a sizable amount of necrosis has taken place.

Medications of use are gabapentin (Neurontin), pregabalin (Lyrica), carbamazepine (Tegretol), nortriptyline (Aventyl, Pamelor), duloxetine (Cymbalta), lamotrigine (Lamictal), and tramadol (Ultram).

56. Travel Concerns

Older adults have more travel concerns than their younger counterparts due to lower immunity, muscle strength, and balance and medication issues. It is recommended that they be more cautious and better preparation for travel.

Older adults wish to visit foreign countries since they have more free time and desire to enjoy their retirement. They also visit friends and families more often as they get older.

Planning is important for successful travel. Older adults should evaluate their level of fitness to be certain that the trip is not strenuous, arrange comfortable seating, and inform the airline of their disabilities, if any. Regular medications should always be in their personal possession and not be packed inside checked luggage. Checked luggage can be lost or delayed. The travel itself may get delayed, and one should not miss their medications at scheduled intervals.

Besides routine medications, one should also pack contingency or emergency items. Such items include allergy pills, antidiarrheal medications, pain medications, heartburn pills, common lozenges, Band-Aids, and tapes.

Travelers need to be aware of the following potential challenges that may occur while traveling:

- Change of time zones
- Change of environment, including pollution
- Food allergies
- Food poisonings
- Hazards associated with walking or other activities
- Fall risks and other dangers
- Risks associated with tours
- Animals
- Availability of toilet facilities
- Drinking water
- Recommended vaccinations
- Skin protections with insect spray or solar lotions
- Proper clothing or hats
- Weather conditions or accommodation-related issues

The whole rhythm of life changes compared to their norm, exposing them to potential dangers. Travelers need to be aware of health-care facilities and medical insurance protections in the area they are traveling.

Long hours of sitting in the same position can cause deep vein thrombosis. Recommendations include walking and stretching every two or three hours. Travelers should avoid physical contact or close contact with strangers or fellow passengers to prevent transmissible infections.

57. Tremors

Tremors can be due to extrapyramidal neurological disorder or related to endocrine disorders. Other causes include anxiety and emotional distress, medication effects, toxemia, and alcohol or drug abuse.

The tremor can be a physiological tremor or essential tremor. Physiological tremors are low amplitude and increased with stress, anxiety, fatigue, toxins, medications, and emotional upsets. They can be coarse or fine tremors, and they can be obvious or subtle. Usually, tremors are noticeable in the hands and fingers but can be seen in lower extremities, tongue, or even head and neck. Essential tremors are familial in 50 percent of cases common in upper extremities, head, and neck and increases with antigravity movements. They are symmetric and high frequency with more flexion-extension tremors. Propranolol or Mysoline are useful.

Cerebellar tremors are short cycles present only during movement, increase with action, and increase in amplitude when a target is reached.

In Parkinson's disease, there is pill-rolling movement at rest, which increases with emotional stress. It is a rhythmic, oscillatory, involuntary movement. It is a slow asymmetric movement with a pronation-supination component to it. In the early stages, tremors appears only when the patient is distracted, as in walking or talking. As the disease progresses, tremors are always obvious. Treatment is with medications further described in chapter 12.

Drugs that cause tremors include amphetamines, antidepressants, antipsychotics, B-agonists, corticosteroids, lithium, amiodarone, methylxanthines (coffee, tea), thyroid hormones, and valproic acid.

58. Varicose Veins

Varicose veins are engorged and visible tortuous veins in the lower extremity that cause cosmetic and medical concerns to the patient. Varicose veins can be primarily due to incompetence of the valves. The valves allow the blood to flow against gravity, and when incompetent, back pressure builds up, and over time, they dilate.

The varicosities can affect the long saphenous system or the short saphenous system. Over time, there is development of pigmentation changes of skin, ulceration, and swelling. Prominent varicosities are treated by surgical stripping and multiple ligations, infrared therapy, or laser therapy. Secondary varicosities are clusters of veins presenting as venous ectasia without involvement of long or short saphenous venous systems. Often, they are postsurgical or due to deep vein thrombosis. They could also be idiopathic. Treatment includes local excision and ligation or sclerotherapy.

Women may present with cosmetic concerns related to spider veins that are visible under the skin on fair skin persons. They do not cause any medical problems and do not require treatment. Alternatively, sclerotherapy or cutaneous laser therapy are options.

59. Vertigo

Vertigo is a spinning sensation that can lead to unsteady gait, nausea, vomiting, and dizziness. The cause can be from middle ear problems, labyrinthitis related to medications, toxemia, or sepsis. Meniere's disease, also known as endolymphatic hydrops, presents with episodic rotational vertigo associated with hearing loss, fullness of ear, and tinnitus.

A common cause of vertigo is benign paroxysmal positional vertigo (BPPV), which is caused by displacement of otoconia (biocrystals comprised of calcium carbonate normally embedded in the saccule and utricle). The displaced material stimulates hair cells in the posterior semicircular canal, creating the sensation of motion. Otitis media, head trauma, Meniere's disease, prolonged anesthesia or bed rest, viral infections, occlusion of anterior vestibular artery, ear surgery, or labyrinthine concussion can trigger this condition. Patients with this condition may experience short periods of vertigo associated with head movements or sitting up, felt more in the early morning hours. These symptoms may be associated with nausea or vomiting, but there is no hearing loss or tinnitus. This form of vertigo can be treated with different maneuvers described as Epley maneuver or Semont maneuver or Brandt-Daroff exercises. All these maneuvers try to reposition the crystals into the utricle by making head rotations and body position changes. They are usually effective. Medications are not needed to treat this type of vertigo.

60. Vomiting

Vomiting is a symptom of an underlying disorder, and the cause can be elucidated through history and physical examination.

Vomiting can be caused by disorders of the gastrointestinal system or related to the central nervous system. Conditions such as acute gastritis, gastric outlet obstruction, pyloric stenosis, intestinal obstruction, or food poisoning are due to local obstructive or inflammatory causes. Conditions such as postanesthetic recovery, drug reactions, sepsis, viral infections, motion sickness, central nervous lesions, and head trauma are due to central origin. Hyperemesis gravidarum is centrally mediated due to pregnancy. Bulimia-induced emesis is related to psychological issues.

Treatment is directed to control symptoms with antiemetics. However, any gastrointestinal obstructive pathology not responding to conservative measures should be corrected with surgical intervention. Nutritional support needs to be addressed as well.

Venkit S. Iyer, MD and David Bernstein, MD

Section 3

Medical Care of
the Older Adult

Chapter 3

Cardiac Care

This chapter describes a limited number of common conditions affecting the older adult. One should refer to cardiology textbooks for detailed discussions on the subject.

The cardiac system contributes to a significant component of the health of the older adult patient, and it contributes to the most common causes of death in this age group.

Atrial fibrillation

Atrial fibrillation is a common cardiac arrhythmia in the older adult, where the atrial contractions are irregular and not followed by ventricular contractions.

Atrial fibrillation has multiple causes such as congestive heart failure, coronary artery disease, valvular disorders, atrial ischemia, hypertension, or neurohumoral cascade. Contributing factors can be sleep disorders, excess use of caffeine, alcohol, or stress. Hyperthyroidism, COPD, or pericardial disease may precipitate the onset of atrial fibrillation.

Atrial fibrillation can be completely asymptomatic for years, or it can be associated with rapid ventricular rate symptomatic with complications, including cardiac failure, stroke, or peripheral emboli from clots in the atria. Patients may experience palpitations, shortness of breath, chest pain, or dizziness.

The diagnosis is determined by observation of irregularly irregular pulse on palpation and irregular heart sounds on auscultation. EKG shows irregular atrial contractions often without identifiable P waves, irregular ventricular contractions, associated changes of old myocardial ischemia, left ventricular hypertrophy, and varying bundle branch blocks.

Transthoracic echocardiogram (TEE) is useful to determine heart size, presence of thrombi in cardiac chambers, valvular disease, and pericardial disease.

Atrial fibrillation is managed with anticoagulants to prevent thromboembolic episodes. Warfarin was the usual anticoagulant. There are now newer and safer medications on the market for this purpose. The major risk of anticoagulation is bleeding, and the concern will be quickness with which they can be reversed in times of emergencies. A review of various drugs, side effects and complications, and the best choice for an individual are made in consultation with a cardiologist. For those who cannot take anticoagulants, two options are available— *watchman* procedure, which is a catheter-based technique to exclude the atrial appendage, or *lariat* epicardial/endocardial suture system to ligate the atrial appendage.

Rapid ventricular rates need to be controlled. Initially, drugs such as digoxin, beta-blockers, calcium channel blockers, or amiodarone are used. The patient may need a pacemaker insertion for node modification.

Cardioversion or ablation therapies are procedures that need careful evaluation with the help of a cardiologist. Identification of precipitating causes and correction of such factors is a vital part in the management of atrial fibrillation.

Table 1

Medications having antithrombotic/anticoagulant effects

Antiplatelets
Aspirin 50–325 mg per day
Dipyridamole (Persantine) 75–100 mg PO, 5 mg IV
Dipyridamole/aspirin (Aggrenox) one tab q twelve hours
Clopidogrel (Plavix) 300–600 mg initially followed by 75 mg daily
Prasugrel (Effient) 60 mg initially followed by 10 mg daily
Ticagrelor (Brilinta) 180 mg initially followed by 90 mg twice daily

Anticoagulants
Heparin (unfractionated) 5,000 units initially followed by twelve to fifteen units per kilogram per hour IV titrated with PTT level
Low-molecular-weight Heparin
Enoxaparin (Lovenox) 40 mg subQ once daily or 1 mg per kilogram q twelve hours
Dalteparin (Fragmin) 2,500–5,000 units subQ once daily or two hundred units per kilogram per day
Tinzaparin (Innohep) 175 units per kilogram per day
Danaparoid (Orgaran) 750 units subQ q twelve hours
Warfarin (Coumadin) 10 mg PO initially and adjust daily dose with daily/weekly INR to keep it in a range of 2 to 3

Factor X-a inhibitors
Apixaban (Eliquis) 5 mg Po q twelve hours

Edoxaban (Savaysa) 60 mg PO once daily
Fondaparinux (Arixtra) 5–10 mg subQ once daily
Rivaroxaban (Xarelto) 10–20 mg PO once daily

Direct thrombin inhibitors
Argatroban 2 mcg/kg/min IV
Bivalirudin (Angiomax) 0.75 mg/kg bolus followed by
1.75 mg/kg IV infusion
Dabigatran (Pradaxa) 15 mg q twelve hours
Desirudin (Iprivask) 15 mg subQ q twelve hours
Lepirudin (Refludan) 4 mg/kg bolus followed by 0.15 mg/kg/hr.

Glycoprotein IIb/IIIa inhibitors
Abciximab (ReoPro) 0.25 mg/kg IV bolus followed by
0.125 mg/kg/minute
Eptifibatide (Integrilin) 180 mcg/kg IV bolus followed by
2 mcg/kg/minute
Tirofiban (Aggrastat) 0.4 mcg/kg/minute over thirty
minutes followed by 0.1 mcg/kg/minute

Table 2

Medications for rhythm control

Amiodarone (Cordarone, Pacerone) 100–200 mg/day
Propafenone (Rythmol) 150–300 mg q eight hours
Sotalol (Betapace, Sorine) 40–160 mg q twelve hours
Adenosine (Adenocard, Adenoscan) 6 mg IV bolus
Quinidine (Quinaglute, Quinora) 200–300 mg q eight hours

For reducing ventricular rate
Metoprolol 2.5–5.00 mg IV bolus
Lopressor (Metoprolol) 100 mg PO q six to twelve hours
Inderal (Propranolol) 1–3 mg IV
Diltiazem (Cardizem) 0.25 mg/kg IV
Verapamil 0.075–0.15 mg/kg IV
Digoxin (Lanoxin, Digitek) 1.25–2.5 mg IV or PO, titrate

For CPR
Adrenaline (Epipen, Adrenaclick) 1 mg (10 ml of 0.1
 mg solution) IV
For hypotension, adrenaline 0.05–2.0 mcg/kg titrate

For symptomatic refractory bradycardia, adrenaline
2–10 mcg/minute

Myocardial infarction

About 1.5 million new cases of acute myocardial infarction occur every year in the USA. It is death of the myocardial muscle tissue due to acute ischemia commonly precipitated by sudden blockage of the coronary artery. Depending upon the location and extent of muscle damage, symptoms vary from silent heart attacks to sudden death.

Symptoms can be as mild as fatigue, chest pain, or malaise. Chest pain is a hallmark. Patients describe it as intense, unrelenting, and suffocating. Substernal pain or discomfort can radiate to the neck, left arm, jaws, and shoulder. The symptoms can be described as a deep squeezing, aching, and burning sensation. At times it is felt in the epigastrium. Other symptoms such as syncope, hypotension, sweating, and shock can occur.

Conditions such as gastrointestinal, pulmonary, musculoskeletal, or neurological disorders can mimic acute coronary syndrome and need to be differentiated.

An initial heart rhythm might be tachycardia and later varying rhythm are detected. It can vary from atrial flutter or atrial fibrillation to ventricular tachycardia or ventricular fibrillation. Hypotension and oliguria can follow. Breathing difficulty, coughing, and frothy sputum followed by pulmonary congestion occurs.

Troponin levels are measured serially. Other blood tests include complete blood count, lipid profile, metabolic profile, and chemistries. CPK-MB levels are elevated. BNP (B-type natriuretic peptide) levels are elevated in the setting of congestive heart failure. EKG changes include elevation of ST segment, Q wave, T wave inversion, and bundle branch block.

Immediate management includes administration of sublingual nitrates, administration of beta-blockers, and pain control with morphine and emergency cardiac resuscitation as needed, including defibrillation if needed.

Decisions are made if there is ST elevation (STEMI) or not. If it is a STEMI, an emergency coronary angiogram is performed to identify the area of blockage. Angioplasty and stent placement are remarkably effective if performed within ninety minutes of onset of symptoms. An alternative option is to give thrombolytic therapy such as TPA or streptokinase if there are no contraindications. Such contraindications would include a history of intracranial bleeding or stroke, brain tumors, history of bleeding disorders, or hemorrhagic conditions.

Medical therapy includes sublingual nitroglycerine, systemic support, beta-blockers, diltiazem, control of hypertension, clopidogrel or aspirin, oxygen bed rest, ReoPro, vasodilators, ACE inhibitors, and PCSK9 inhibitors such as evolocumab, and pain control with morphine. Potassium and magnesium levels are monitored and maintained in a normal range.

Post-MI management includes cessation of smoking, control of cholesterol and lipids, aspirin, anticoagulation, cardiac rehabilitation to include diet, exercise, and stress reduction, management of hypertension, and use of other cardiac medications as recommended by the cardiologist.

Table 3

Medications for dyslipidemia

Statins
Atorvastatin (Lipitor) 10–80 mg per day
Fluvastatin (Lescol, Lescol XL) 20–80 mg per day
Pitavastatin (Livalol) 1–4 mg per day
Pravastatin (Pravachol) 10–80 mg per day
ASA/Pravachol (Pravigard) one tab per day
Rosuvastatin (Crestor, Ezalor) 5–40 mg per day
Simvastatin (Zocor) 10–40 mg per day
Lovastatin (Mevacor, Altoprev) 10–40 mg per day

Fibrates
Fenofibrate (Tricor, Lofibra, Antara) 48–200 mg per day
Fenofibrate delayed release (Triplix) 45–135 mg per day
Gemfibrozil (Lopid) 300–600 mg q twelve hours

Cholesterol absorption inhibitor
Ezetimibe (Zetia) 10 mg per day
Nicotinic acid (no longer considered effective)
Niacin 100 mg to 1,000 mg q eight hours
Niacin ER (Niaspan) 500–2,000 mg per day

Bile acid sequestrant

Cholestyramine (Questran, Questran Light) 4 mg daily
Colesevelam (Welchol) 1,850 to 3,750 mg per day
Colestipol (Colestid) 5–30 mg per day

Fatty acids
Omega-3 acid (Omacor, Lovaza) 4 mg per day
Icosapent ethyl (Vascepa) 1 mg two capsules twice daily

Combinations
Ezetimibe/Simvastatin (Vytorin) 10–40 mg per day
Lovastatin/Niacin (Advicor) 20–40 mg per day
(*no longer considered effective*)
Simvastatin/Niacin (Simcor) 20–40 mg per day
(*no longer considered effective*)

PCSK9 inhibitor
Alirocumab (Praluent) 75–150 mg subQ q two weeks
Evolocumab (Repatha) 140 mg every two weeks

Newer drug
Nexletol (Bempedoic acid) 180 mg once daily PO

Angina pectoris

About 9.8 million people experience angina symptoms every year in the USA. It is a symptom of myocardial ischemia presenting as retrosternal discomfort, chest pain, or exertional pain. The most common cause of angina is atherosclerotic heart disease. Other causes include cardiomyopathy and mitral valve disease. There is vascular spasm even when there is no fixed obstructive lesion. Unstable angina could be due to a platelet thrombus.

Initially, angina presents as chest pain induced by exercise and relieved by nitroglycerin. Subsequently, it can lead to a myocardial infarction.

Exercise stress test, thallium stress test, and coronary calcium scoring with fast CT are initial tests of value. Subsequently, a coronary angiogram is performed to better evaluate the coronary anatomy.

Initial management of angina includes cessation of smoking and reduction of LDL and lipoproteins. Further management includes pharmacological agents such as aspirin, clopidogrel, beta-blockers, calcium channel blockers, and ACE inhibitors. Recent large-scale studies show that stent placements or coronary bypass procedures are unnecessary for asymptomatic or mildly symptomatic angina patients. Lifestyle changes such as diet, exercise, and medications are effective. Interventions are appropriate only for very severe stenosis with symptoms. Severe cases with coronary stenosis are candidates for angioplasty and stent placement or aortocoronary bypass procedure.

Table 4

Medication list of nitrites

Oral
Isosorbide dinitrate (Isordil, Sorbitrate)10–40 mg three times a day
Isosorbide dinitrate SR (Dilatrate SR) 40–80 mg q eight hours
Isosorbide mononitrate (ISMO, Monoket) 20 mg q twelve hours
Isosorbide mononitrate SR (Imdur) 30–60 mg per day
Nitroglycerine (Nitro Bid) 2.5–9 mg q eight hours

Sublingual
Isosorbide dinitrate (Isordil, Sorbitrate) 5 mg tablets
Nitroglycerine (Nitrostat, Nitroquick) 0.3–0.6 mg tab

Oral spray
Nitroglycerine (Nitro Mist, Nitrolingual)

Ointment
Nitroglycerine 2 percent

Transdermal
Nitroglycerine (Nitro Patch, Minitran) 0.1 mg/hr to 0.8 mg/hr

---

Congestive heart failure (CHF)

CHF is the accumulation of interstitial fluid in the pulmonary parenchyma due to increased pulmonary venous pressure occurring because of cardiac dysfunction. The interference with oxygen exchange leads to dyspnea, anxiety, fatigue, tachycardia, tissue edema, distended neck veins, rales and rhonchi, cyanosis, ascites, hepatomegaly and arrhythmias, cardiac failure, and death.

The etiology could be due to atrial outflow obstruction caused by mitral stenosis, atrial myxoma, or thrombosis of the prosthetic valve. The cause could be due to left ventricular dysfunction as in myocardial infarction, myocarditis, chronic cardiac valvular disease, severe anemia, nutritional, toxins, and noncompliance with medications or thyrotoxicosis. Left ventricular volume overload can be extrinsic or intrinsic.

A physical examination reveals tachycardia, tachypnea, pulmonary rales, distended jugulars, edema of legs or dependent tissue edema, and hepatomegaly. Associated conditions such as hypertension, valvular disorders, pericarditis, or renal disorders may contribute.

The differential diagnosis between cardiogenic and noncardiogenic pulmonary edema is necessary since conditions such as pneumothorax, high-altitude pulmonary edema, neurogenic pulmonary edema, allergic reaction, asthma, chronic obstructive pulmonary disease, and bacterial and viral pneumonia can mimic congestive heart failure.

The heart suffers from diminished ability to respond to stress with advancing age. There is a reduced responsiveness to beta-adrenergic stimulation, increased vascular stiffness leading to increased afterload, increased cardiac stiffness leading to decreased diastolic filling, and decreased mitochondrial ability to respond to ATP demands.

Echocardiogram shows dilated ventricles. EKG shows LV dysfunction. Chest x-ray shows cardiomegaly and fluid in the lung parenchyma, and noninvasive stress test shows ischemic myocardium. Treatment includes fluid restriction to avoid fluid overload, judicious use of diuretics, control of hypertension, digoxin, management of diabetes and hyperlipidemia, moderate salt restriction, and avoidance of exertion.

Hypertension (HTN)

High blood pressure (HTN) can be primary, also known as essential hypertension, or secondary due to other causative factors. Over 50 percent of the population above the age of sixty-five has hypertension. Both systolic and diastolic levels are to be considered in diagnosing hypertension. Systolic pressure above 140 and diastolic pressure above 80 meets the criteria for the diagnosis of hypertension and requires medical attention.

A causative factor is atherosclerosis with decreased elasticity of blood vessels, leading to increased peripheral vascular resistance. Other causative factors are diabetes mellitus, obesity, smoking, and medication effects, endocrine disorders such as pheochromocytoma, primary hyperaldosteronism, Cushing's syndrome, renal diseases, renal artery stenosis, and dietary habits.

In the early stages, HTN is asymptomatic. As the problem worsens, various effects occur, such as hypertensive heart disease, congestive heart failure, stroke, retinal hemorrhage, renal insufficiency, and hypertensive crisis. Keeping the blood pressure in normal range helps preserve good health.

Investigations include routine blood tests and lipid profile and evaluation of renal functions. High blood pressure needs an endocrine work up. EKG and chest x-rays are performed for baseline status. Blood pressure must be checked in both upper extremities for follow-up. Other special investigations such as CT scan, MRI, or angiograms are ordered on a case-by-case basis to detect any other reversible cause of HTN.

Nonpharmacological treatments include regular exercise, stress reduction, and reduction in dietary salt intake, smoking cessation, reduced alcohol intake, and avoidance of NSAIDs. A variety of medications are available for treating hypertension. A carefully planned long-term approach is necessary when starting the drug regimen and follow up.

Table 5

Medications for hypertension

Diuretics
Thiazides:
Chlorothiazide (Diuril) 125–500 mg/day
Chlorthalidone (Hygroton) 12.5–25 mg/day
Hydrochlorothiazide (HCTZ, Microzide) 12.5–25 mg/day
Indapamide (Lozol) 0.625–2.5 mg/day
Metolazone (Zaroxolyn, Mykrox) 2.5–5.0 mg/day
Polythiazide (Renese) 1–4 mg/day

Loop diuretics:
Bumetanide (Bumex) 0.5–4 mg/day
Furosemide (Lasix) 20–160 mg/day
Torsemide (Demadex) 2.5–50 mg/day

Potassium sparing:
Amiloride (Midamor) 2.5–10 mg/day
Triamterene (Dyrenium) 25–100 mg/day

Hydrochlorothiazide/Triamterene (Maxzide, Dyazide) 25 mg/ 37.5 mg

Aldosterone receptor blockers:
Eplerenone (Inspra) 25–100 mg/day
Spironolactone (Aldactone, Carospir) 12.5–25 mg/day

Adrenergic inhibitors
Alpha-1 blockers:
Doxazosin (Cardura) 1–16 mg/day
Prazosin (Minipress) 1–20 mg/day
Terazosin (Hytrin) 1–20 mg/day

Central alpha 2 agonists:
Clonidine (Catapres) 0.1–1.2 mg/day
Guanfacine (Tenex) 05–2 mg/day
Methyldopa (Aldomet) 250–2,500 mg/day
Reserpine (Serpasil) 0.05–0.25 mg/day

Beta blockers:
Acebutolol (Sectral) 200–800 mg/day
Atenolol (Tenormin) 12.5–100 mg/day
Betaxolol (Kerlone) 5–20 mg/day
Bisoprolol (Zebeta) 2.5–10 mg/day
Metoprolol (Lopressor) 25–400 mg/day
Nadolol (Corgard) 20–160 mg/day
Nebivolol (Bystolic) 2.5–40 mg/day
Penbutolol (Levatol) 10–40 mg/day
Pindolol (Visken) 5–40 mg/day
Propranolol (Inderal) 20–160 mg/day
Timolol (Blocarden) 10–40 mg/day

Combined alpha and beta blockers:
Carvedilol (Coreg) 3.125–25 mg/day
Labetalol (Normodyne, Trandate)100–600 mg/day

Vasodilators:
Hydralazine (Apresoline) 25–100 mg/day
Minoxidil (Loniten) 2.5–50 mg/day

Calcium channel blockers/antagonists:

Nondihydropyridines
Diltiazem (Cardizem) 120–360 mg/day
Verapamil (Calan, Isoptin, Verelan) 120–360 mg/day

Dihydropyridines:
Amlodipine (Norvasc) 2.5–10 mg/day
Felodipine (Plendil) 2.5–20 mg/day
Isradipine (Dynacirc) 2.5–10 mg/day
Nicardipine (Cardene) 60–120 mg/day
Nifedipine (Adalat, Procardia)30–60 mg/day
Nisoldipine (Sular) 10–40 mg/day

ACE inhibitors:
Benazepril (Lotensin) 2.5–40 mg/day
Captopril (Capoten) 12.5–150 mg/day
Enalapril (Vasotec) 2.5–40 mg/day
Fosinopril (Monopril) 5–40 mg/day
Lisinopril (Prinivil, Zestril) 2.5–40 mg/day
Moexipril (Univasc) 3.75–40 mg/day
Perindopril (Aceon) 4–8 mg/day
Quinapril (Accupril) 5–40 mg/day
Ramipril (Altace) 1.25–20 mg/day
Trandolapril (Mavik) 1–4 mg/day
Accuretic/Quinaretic (Quinapril with Hydrochlorothiazide) 10–20 mg with 12.5 mg HCTZ
Amlodipine besylate / benazepril (Lotrel) 10 mg / 2.5 mg to 40 mg /10 mg

ARBs (angiotensin II receptor blockers):
Azilsartan (Edarbi) 20–80 mg/day
Candesartan (Atacand) 4–32 mg/day
Eprosartan (Teveten) 400–800 mg/day
Irbesartan (Avapro) 75–300 mg/day
Losartan (Cozaar) 12.5–100 mg/day
Olmesartan (Benicar) 20–40 mg/day
Telmisartan (Micardis) 20–80 mg/day
Valsartan (Diovan) 40–320 mg/day

Renin inhibitor:
Aliskiren (Tekturna) 150–300 mg/day

For rapid control of hypertension by intravenous route, for conditions such as hypertensive encephalopathy, dissecting aneurysm of aorta, postoperative carotid endarterectomy, LVH with pulmonary edema, adrenergic crisis, malignant hypertension, and acute renal failure:

Nitroglycerine drip
Nitroprusside drip
Labetalol
Captopril
Minoxidil
Propranolol

Aortic valve disease in the older adult

As populations continue to age, aortic stenosis becomes the most prevalent valvular disease in Western countries. The number of older patients with aortic stenosis continues to pose both diagnostic and therapeutic challenges. Despite new advances such as transcatheter aortic valve replacement (TAVR), there is still considerable patient-provider decision-making necessary, given the comorbidities and complex goals of care in the aging patient population.

Increased longevity from advances in health care has resulted in an increase in diagnosis of aortic stenosis. While the prevalence is low in patients younger than sixty years of age, it increases to approximately 10 percent in patients older than eighty years of age. The severity of aortic stenosis increases with age, with one in eight people older than age seventy-five showing moderate to severe aortic stenosis. Among symptomatic patients with medically treated moderate-to-severe aortic stenosis, mortality from the onset of symptoms is approximately 25 percent at one year and 50 percent at two years.

Aortic stenosis represents a significant healthcare burden and with our aging society cases and intervention are projected to increase significantly. Clinical risk factors for degenerative aortic valve stenosis mirror those associated with coronary atherosclerosis. The development and progression of aortic stenosis has been associated with traditional cardiovascular risk factors such as age, male gender, smoking, elevated LDL cholesterol, hypertension, and metabolic syndrome.

In evaluating elderly patients with aortic stenosis, it is important to elicit a comprehensive and meticulous history. The three cardinal symptoms of aortic stenosis that prompt urgent valve replacement include angina, syncope, and heart failure symptoms (including orthopnea, edema, and paroxysmal nocturnal dyspnea). In this population, it is difficult to elicit symptoms as these individuals have significantly decreased mobility or might not be aware of their symptoms.

The following studies are components in the diagnosis and assessment of aortic stenosis:

- Serum electrolyte levels
- Cardiac biomarkers
- Complete blood count
- B-type natriuretic peptide (provides incremental prognostic information for predicting symptom onset in asymptomatic patients with severe aortic stenosis; increased levels are associated with aortic stenosis-related adverse events in asymptomatic severe aortic stenosis)
- Electrocardiography (ECG) (serial ECG can show the progression of aortic stenosis)
- Chest radiography
- Echocardiography (two-dimensional and Doppler)
- Cardiac catheterization (based on clinical findings inconsistent with echocardiogram results)
- Coronary angiography
- Radionuclide ventriculography (may provide information on left ventricular function)
- Exercise stress testing (contraindicated in symptomatic patients with severe aortic stenosis)

Transthoracic echocardiography (TTE) remains the gold standard for evaluating aortic stenosis. Clinicians should not depend solely on the echocardiogram for clinical decision-making. It is imperative that the clinician connect the history, physical findings, and imaging results.

When evaluating risk, it is important to evaluate frailty, disability, mobility, cognitive impairment, nutritional status, and fall risk. Shared clinician-patient decision-making is equally important.

Frailty is defined as a state of vulnerability, a syndrome characterized by decreased physiological reserve and diminished resistance to stressors. Despite the significant comorbidities of the elderly, the outcomes for aortic valve replacement have been improving.

Aortic stenosis has high morbidity and mortality after the occurrence of symptoms, where the two-year mortality risk is higher than 50 percent. Aortic valve replacement with either open-heart surgery or TAVR are the only treatment modalities that reduce morbidity and mortality with significant aortic stenosis. Percutaneous balloon valvuloplasty is used as a palliative measure in critically ill adult patients who are not surgical candidates or as a bridge to aortic valve replacement in those critically ill patients.

Pericardial disease

Pericardial effusion can put pressure on the heart, affecting how the heart works. If untreated, it may lead to heart failure or death in extreme cases. Pericardial effusions may not cause any noticeable signs and symptoms, particularly if the fluid has increased slowly.

If pericardial effusion signs and symptoms do occur, they might include the following:

- Shortness of breath or difficulty breathing
- Discomfort when breathing while lying down
- Chest pain usually behind the breastbone or on the left side of the chest
- Chest fullness
- Lightheadedness or feeling faint
- Swelling in the abdomen or legs

Pericardial disease with an effusion results from the inflammation of the pericardium after an illness or injury. In the case of an older adult, effusions are often discovered to be associated with cancers. There are cases of idiopathic pericarditis when the cause cannot be determined.

Causes of pericardial effusion may include the following:

- Autoimmune disorders such as rheumatoid arthritis or lupus
- Cancer of the heart or pericardium
- Spread of cancer (metastasis), particularly lung cancer, breast cancer, or Hodgkin's lymphoma
- Radiation therapy for cancer if the heart was exposed to radiation
- Chest trauma
- Inflammation of the pericardium following a heart attack, heart surgery, or a procedure where the heart's lining is injured
- Underactive thyroid (hypothyroidism)
- Use of certain drugs or exposure to toxins
- Viral, bacterial, fungal, or parasitic infections
- Kidney failure (uremia)
- Constrictive pericarditis with thickened fibrotic inelastic pericardium restricting the function of the heart

A potential complication of pericardial effusion is cardiac tamponade. The strain from the effusion and tamponade prevents the heart chambers from filling completely with blood, resulting in poor blood flow and a lack of oxygen in the body. Cardiac tamponade is life-threatening and requires emergency medical treatment.

Treatment requires the drainage of the effusion via a percutaneous approach or via surgical intervention with a pericardial window.

Pacemaker/AICD issues

It is estimated that worldwide, three million people have pacemakers implanted, with about 600,000 procedures done each year. Most pacemakers are implanted in patients over age sixty.

Pacemakers ensure a minimum number of heartbeats when situations arise where the heartbeat is slow or inadequate. Usual indications are conduction system abnormalities such as in second- and third-degree heart blocks, long sinus pauses, the necessity of taking medications that reduce heart rate, congestive heart failure, congenital heart disease, heart transplantation, prior heart attacks, and atrial fibrillation requiring ablation therapy. With advances in medical technology, distinct types of pacemakers are implanted, such as single-chamber, dual-chamber, biventricular, and wireless pacers. Patients require periodic monitoring and precautions in care of the pacemaker.

Ethical and moral questions can arise from patients with end-of-life issues relating to the maintenance of pacemakers.

AICD stands for automatic implantable cardioverter defibrillator, which is another implanted device for patients who are at substantial risk for ventricular tachycardia or ventricular fibrillation resulting in sudden death. This can happen in individuals who had prior myocardial infarction or with low ejection fraction of less than 30 percent and severe cardiomyopathy.

Even though cardiologists are the best-suited specialists in the care of these devices, it is relevant for geriatricians to know about these devices since AICDs are typically implanted in older adults.

Chapter 4

Stroke

The second most common cause of death and disability for the older adult is stroke. It is a sudden cerebrovascular accident usually due to atherosclerotic disease or embolic events resulting in hemiplegia and aphasia, leading to various morbidities and death. Other causes of stroke are trauma with head injuries, intracranial bleeding secondary to diseases, aneurysms, uncontrolled hypertension, tumors, or medications such as anticoagulants. Congenital disorders and cancer conditions, infections, metabolic problems leading to encephalopathy, meningitis, and certain parasitic infestations can also cause strokes.

Risk factors for stroke include diabetes mellitus, hypertension, atherosclerotic peripheral vascular disease, coronary artery disease, history of myocardial infarction, atrial fibrillation, smoking, hyperlipidemia, homocysteinemia, falls, and anticoagulants.

Chronic atherosclerotic plaque buildup can occur at the carotid artery bifurcation or in other major arteries. These plaques can progressively get larger and eventually occlude the lumen. They can cause turbulence and function as a focal point for platelet thrombi to form, which can break off and occlude the middle cerebral artery or other intracranial vessels. Another possibility is that the plaques themselves break off and go downstream as atherosclerotic emboli and occlude the distal lumen.

Emboli can arise from the heart itself. Mural thrombi can arise in the atrial appendage related to atrial fibrillation, valvular diseases, aneurysmal diseases, or atrial myxoma. Air emboli or fat emboli can also function as emboli resulting in anoxic brain damage.

Many patients experience a set of symptoms described as transient ischemic attacks (TIA). They are considered as mini strokes or warning signs of an impending full-blown stroke. They occur because of microemboli entering the cerebrovascular system. Such symptoms include transient weakness of one limb or one side of the body with recovery, sudden dizziness or syncopal episode, transient blindness of one eye (known as amaurosis fugax), sudden slurring of speech, or sudden unexplained fall.

Once a full stroke occurs, anoxic brain damage takes place to one side or one part of the brain. Right side carotid artery occlusion causes the right side of the brain to suffer, which controls the left side of the body, thus leading to left side hemiplegia. The left cerebral hemisphere controls the right side of the body and the speech center. Thus, left hemispheric ischemia causes aphasia in addition to right hemiplegia. Sometimes there are only microemboli causing minimal damage to brain tissue. There is excellent cross collateral circulation through the circle of Willis, which can protect the entire brain even if one of the carotid arteries is completely blocked/occluded.

Other causes of stroke include intracranial hemorrhage. One can develop intracranial patchy hemorrhage, or it can be an extradural or subdural hematoma from trauma. Subarachnoid hemorrhage is often spontaneous. Gunshot wounds cause extensive brain damage. Falls and blunt trauma can cause brain congestion. One can also develop intracranial blood vessel thrombosis due to extensive peripheral atherosclerosis.

Initial testing would include carotid duplex scan by ultrasound modality. One can measure the flow velocity and extent of narrowing of the artery by this test. A CT scan of the head or an MRI scan of the brain are typically ordered to study the extent of brain damage and etiology. Changes can be progressive and may take days to evolve; hence serial scans are compared over a period of several days. One will have to consider doing an emergency cerebral angiogram. These tests are performed with the goal of therapy, such as immediate administration of thrombolytic or doing other endovascular or open surgical interventions.

If there is evidence of carotid artery stenosis for over 80 percent or over 70 percent with symptoms of TIA, then one should consider prophylactic carotid endarterectomy. Those who are unsuitable for surgery are candidates for endovascular angioplasty and stent placement. All patients are also placed on aspirin or clopidogrel. Smoking cessation is strongly recommended and along with aggressive cholesterol and lipid control.

Once an acute cerebrovascular accident occurs, urgent intervention and treatment within a brief window of three hours offers the patient the best possible outcome. This involves urgent carotid ultrasound, CT scan, or MRI to rule out brain tumors or intracranial bleeding. Treatment with thrombolytics such as TPA are infused, and additional endovascular interventions considered if necessary. Stroke teams have been set up in most major hospitals to provide prompt intervention and treatment. If successfully done, these rapid response measures give the best potential for recovery.

Once a stroke is recognized, and the golden period of sixty to ninety minutes for interventions is over, all one can hope for is natural recovery.

Appropriate investigations include a CT scan or an MRI scan to rule out other causes, such as intracranial bleeding or subdural hematoma or brain cancers. Poststroke management includes physical therapy, speech therapy, and rehabilitation. Efforts to avoid complications, such as contractures, bedsores, urinary tract infections, fractures of long bones, and pneumonia are important. Nutritional support, swallowing studies to enable prevention of aspiration, and psychological and social support are important management considerations. Further, management of comorbidities such as hypertension, diabetes mellitus, and chronic renal insufficiency are included in a treatment plan. Evaluation of the opposite carotid artery for any stenosis is performed to consider the extent of obstruction. A prophylactic carotid endarterectomy is a possibility once the stroke is stable for three months. Patients can recover a good part of the body function with perseverance and effort.

Table 6

Treatments of value in stroke

Thrombotic conditions
Antiplatelets:
Aspirin, Plavix

Anticoagulants:
Heparin, Coumadin

Thrombolytics:
TPA, ReoPro

Brain edema
Mannitol
Steroids
Diamox (Acetazolamide) 8–30 mg/kg/day

Hemorrhagic conditions:
Avoid anticoagulants and thrombolytics
Manage hypertension
Decompression steps
Seizure, agitation, delirium management
Dilantin (Phenytoin, Phenytek) 3–100 mg PO, 15–20 mg/kg

IV/IM

Physical therapy, speech therapy, nutritional support, occupational therapy, respiratory care, DVT precautions, decubitus care, aspiration prevention, bladder and bowel care, and social support in all cases.

Chapter 5

Peripheral Vascular Disorders

Older adults have a higher chance of developing severe peripheral vascular disorders because of increased chance of atherosclerotic lesions with advancing age. These can manifest in the form of pain in the legs and difficulty in walking as intermittent claudication and rest pain or as nonhealing wounds or even as overt gangrene of the extremity. Another manifestation could be abdominal aortic aneurysm and other aneurysms in the body. Finally, diabetic neuropathy and small vessel disease can cause sudden onset of necrotizing soft tissue infections and tissue loss.

Ischemic peripheral vascular disease (PAD)

Ischemic peripheral vascular disease is the most common reason for gangrene of lower extremities. Atherosclerosis is a generalized process and can affect any artery in the body. Plaque buildup occurs at major bifurcations due to turbulence of blood flow. Thus, it occurs often at carotid bifurcation, aortic bifurcation to iliac arteries, common femoral artery where it divides into profunda femoris, and superficial femoral artery and at the trifurcation of the tibial vessels. The manifestation can be slowly progressing ischemic signs and symptoms or sudden exacerbation with acute ischemic changes.

The superficial femoral artery is one of the first vessels to get narrow, irregular, and to occlude in the lower extremity. By itself, it causes very minor problems if the remaining vessels are patent. The collaterals from profunda femoris keep the leg viable. It takes a second level of obstruction somewhere in the arterial tree for the ischemic symptoms to appear.

One of the earliest symptoms of PAD is intermittent claudication. Patients develop pain in the calf muscles upon walking, and resting relieves the pain. It is due to ischemia of the muscles that require augmented blood supply during exercise. Progressively the claudication distance shortens, and eventually there is pain all the time. Rest pain is felt in the calf as well as in the foot, and it can be slightly improved by hanging the leg down. As it further worsens, gangrene of the toes occurs, and small injuries or cuts lead to nonhealing wounds. Eventually the gangrene spreads, requiring below-knee or above-knee amputation.

During an examination, one should ask about a history of smoking, diabetes mellitus, hyperlipidemia, hypertension, scleroderma or other vasculitis conditions, and exposure to trauma or extreme weather conditions. Physical examination must include palpation of all peripheral pulses, evaluation of nails and skin conditions, and evidence of ischemic changes or infections in the affected extremity. Evaluation of atherosclerotic disease elsewhere in the body must be made specifically to assess cardiac condition and carotid artery disease.

One of the simple tests to evaluate for the presence of PAD is measuring the ankle-brachial index. Normally, the blood pressure is the same in upper and lower extremities. Claudication occurs when the AB ratio is less than 0.5, and rest pain occurs when it is 0.25. Low AB ratio should trigger an evaluation for other systemic atherosclerotic problems, such as coronary artery or carotid artery stenosis.

Arterial and venous ultrasound studies with flow velocities are noninvasive and inexpensive tests. An ultrasound can provide valuable information about the arterial and venous status of the lower limbs. Level of occlusion, extent of disease, extent of vascularity, presence of clots in the graft and in the venous system, and patency of grafts and blood vessels can be assessed.

The next test would be an MR angiogram, which is noninvasive, or a CT angiogram that involves injection of a small amount of contrast. Both these tests can be performed as outpatient procedures with minimal complications. They give a valuable view of the arterial channels across the body and from which further management decisions can be made. A final test will be a contrast injected digital angiogram focusing on the problem at hand. This can be combined with any endovascular interventions or as the final road map for any surgical interventions.

Acute arterial obstruction by emboli causes sudden onset of symptoms of severe pain, paresthesia, paralysis, pallor, and absence of a pulse. Treatment can be by open embolectomy or intra-arterial thrombolytic therapy followed by anticoagulation.

Chronic slowly progressive obstructions from atherosclerotic lesions are corrected with angioplasty and/or stent placement, but some might need open surgical procedures. Occasionally the obstructed artery may be repaired by endarterectomy or require a bypass procedure to bring blood from a level above the obstruction to a level below the obstruction. Such bypass procedure can be aorto-bifemoral bypass, iliofemoral bypass, cross femoral bypass, femoral-popliteal bypass, femoral-tibial bypass, distal vessel bypass, or axillofemoral bypass, depending upon the circumstances and anatomy.

Aneurysms

An aneurysm is ballooning of the artery in a certain area, resulting from weakening of the muscle wall of the blood vessel. Common locations are abdominal aorta, thoracic aorta, iliac artery, femoral artery, popliteal artery, visceral arteries, and intracranial arteries. The older population should be concerned about abdominal aortic aneurysm (AAA).

An AAA is asymptomatic until it ruptures. It causes excruciating and unrelenting back pain when it ruptures. Rupture of the AAA is associated with severe blood loss, hemorrhagic shock, hypotension, oliguria, and high chance for death. The natural course of any aneurysm is to expand and eventually rupture without intervention.

The best screening test for an AAA is an abdominal ultrasound. The AAA is easy to see as a localized ballooning of the aorta with normal appearing arteries above and below. The size of the aneurysm can be measured, and relationship to the renal arteries and iliac arteries can be assessed. An infrarenal aortic aneurysm is considered as small when it is 4 cm in size, medium when it becomes 5 cm in size, and large when it becomes 6 cm in size. A CT scan is done to further evaluate the size of the aneurysm to plan further management.

Elective repair of the AAA is recommended to avoid future rupture of the aneurysm. The options to consider are either endovascular stent placement, or open surgery. Both have their merits and drawbacks. For the older adults, endovascular repair (EVAR) is preferable since it can be done under spinal anesthesia or minimal anesthesia. Ambulation and recovery are faster; blood loss and surgical dissections are minimal. In the open repair, the aneurysmal sac is laid open, and a synthetic graft is sewn between the upper end and the lower end of the sac. For the younger patients, an open repair is felt to be better with a favorable long-term outcome.

Popliteal aneurysms can be bilateral and cause distal embolization and sudden occlusion of the trifurcation, resulting in acute onset ischemia of the leg. Popliteal aneurysm can result in amputation unless emergency revascularization surgery is performed.

Visceral aneurysms can rupture spontaneously and result in massive internal hemorrhage. Intracranial aneurysms can cause massive subarachnoid hemorrhage and death. Diagnosis must be made by contrast studies. Visceral aneurysms are often detected as incidental findings during other investigations. Prophylactic surgery to clip or embolize them is recommended.

Deep vein thrombosis (DVT)

Deep vein thrombosis is a problem of concern to the older adult. Clots form spontaneously in the deep veins in the calf muscle areas. Usually, the initiating cause is stasis and immobility. The calf muscles during the muscle contractions push the blood up toward the heart. As the patient is sitting or lying down for long hours due to locomotor problems or illnesses, stasis of blood occurs, which in turn leads to deep vein thrombosis or DVT. Patients complain of pain in the calf muscle area, and there is unilateral edema of the leg. There is evidence of calf tenderness. Homan's sign is positive. Homan's sign is elicitation of pain in the calf area upon flexing the knee and then dorsiflexion of the ankle. The best diagnostic test is an ultrasound of the deep veins. The treatment is to anticoagulate immediately to prevent the clots moving into the pulmonary system that can cause pulmonary emboli. In selected patients who cannot take anticoagulation, one can insert a vena cava filter percutaneously to prevent pulmonary embolism.

Chronic venous insufficiency (DVI)

Deep vein insufficiency is a chronic condition that results in lymphedema of the leg. The valves in the deep vein are defective either from prior thrombophlebitis or from unknown reasons. The blood stagnates in the lower extremity since it must move up against gravity. This leads to chronic swelling, secondary varicosities, chronic induration and pigmentation of tissues, chronic lymphedema, dryness of skin, skin ulcerations, and elephantiasis. Sudden loss of skin occurs from secondary subcutaneous soft tissue infections, which leads to weeping, nonhealing large open wounds. Patients are advised to avoid dryness of the skin and to avoid scratching. The use of moisturizing solutions and creams are helpful. Elevation of the legs and use of ace bandages or tissue compressors are helpful. There is a tendency to recommend surgery to remove the visible secondary varicosities; however, this does not correct the underlying problem. Lymphedema can result from chronic venous insufficiency or from primary lymphatic obstructive disorders, either congenital or acquired.

Table 7

Medications of value in peripheral vascular problems

Antiplatelets:
Aspirin, Plavix
Trental
Anticoagulants for acute thrombi or emboli
Heparin, Coumadin

Antibiotics for infections:
Broad-spectrum coverage
Staph and strep coverage

Topical agents:
Moisturizing creams—hydrogel
Antiseptic agents—silver nitrate
Antibiotic creams—bacitracin, Polysporin, mupirocin
Occlusive dressings—DuoDERM, Opsite

Control of diabetes mellitus, hypertension, vitamin deficiency, antismoking agents, prevention of falls, and trauma.

Venkit S. Iyer, MD and David Bernstein, MD

Chapter 6

Pulmonary Conditions
Chronic Obstructive Pulmonary Disease (COPD)

One of the common respiratory problems affecting older adults is chronic obstructive pulmonary disease. It is a combination of conditions that restrict lung function and oxygen exchange. It is the fourth leading cause of death. Smoking is a major contributing factor. Bronchial asthma, emphysema, tuberculosis, sarcoidosis, obesity, and atmospheric pollution are other contributory factors. Other risk factors are environmental or occupational pollutants, alpha-1 antitrypsin deficiency, childhood history of recurrent respiratory infections, low socioeconomic status, advancing age, and secondhand smoking exposure.

There is decreased elastic recoil of alveoli leading to collapsed airways, and as a result, air exchange is reduced, chest wall compliance is decreased, and vital capacity and FEV1 are decreased. There is evidence of chronic bronchitis, recurrent pulmonary infections, coughing, shortness of breath, wheezing, sputum production, and asthma. This leads to difficulty in walking and as a result, there is a reduction in quality of life and ability to work.

Physical examination shows diminished or distant breath sounds, barrel-shaped chest, hyperresonance on percussion, and prolonged expiratory phase or wheezing. In advanced stages, use of accessory muscles in respiration and distended jugular veins are noted.

Advanced stages lead to pulmonary hypertension, cor pulmonale, cyanosis, peripheral edema, and hepatomegaly. Emphysematous bullae can form, which can rupture, leading to spontaneous pneumothorax.

Chest x-ray shows increased bronchial markings, thinned-out alveolar markings, hyperinflation of lungs, and/or cardiomegaly. PaO2 levels are decreased, FEV1 is lowered, and respiratory acidosis can occur.

Treatment includes total cessation of smoking and avoidance of allergens. Avoid pollution from air and inhalants. Bronchodilator therapy is helpful for symptomatic improvement. Graduated respiratory physical therapy includes exercises, breathing techniques, and moisturized inhalants. Beta-adrenergic agonists and anticholinergic agents are effective in acute episodes of asthma. Ipratropium and Tiotropium are useful. Decongestants and mucosal sputum loosening agents are of marginal benefit. Eventually, corticosteroids are necessary along with respiratory support with CPAP or BIPAP. Persistent airflow obstruction eventually becomes resistant to bronchodilators. Roflumilast is a phosphodiesterase-4 inhibitor, which aims to reduce inflammation by inhibiting breakdown of intracellular cyclic ATP. Exacerbation of acute infections may need antibiotics and oxygen therapy. Bullectomy and lung volume reduction surgery have been used in selected patients.

Prevention includes cessation of all smoking and prophylactic vaccine against influenza and pneumococcal infections.

Table 8

Medications for coughing—antitussives and expectorants

Benzonatate (Tessalon Perles) 100 mg PO q eight hours
Dextromethorphan (Robitussin DM) 10–30 ml PO q four to eight hours
Guaifenesin (Robitussin) 5–20 ml PO q four hours
Codeine phosphate / guaifenesin 10 mg / 100 mg
Hydrocodone/homatropine (Hycodan) 5 ml/q four to six hours
Nasal ipratropium (Atrovent NS) 0.06 percent, two sprays q twelve hours
Pseudoephedrine (decongestant) 60 mg PO q four to six hours
Diphenhydramine 25–50 mg PO q four to six hours
Mucomyst
Dayquil (acetaminophen, dextromethorphan, phenylephrine)
Nyquil (acetaminophen, dextromethorphan, doxylamine)
Theraflu (acetaminophen, pheniramine maleate, phenylephrine)
Chlorpheniramine maleate, dextromethorphan, and phenylephrine hydrochloride
Tylenol plus (acetaminophen, dextromethorphan, guaifenesin, and phenylephrine)

Antihistamines:
Loratadine (Claritin) 10 mg/day
Fexofenadine (Allegra)180 mg/day
Levocetirizine (Xyzal) 2.5 mg po/day
Cetirizine (Zyrtec) 5–10 mg/day
Azelastine nasal spray, one spray q twelve hours
Olopatadine (Patanase) two sprays q twelve hours

Nasal steroids one to two sprays/day
Fluticasone propionate
Fluticasone furoate (Veramyst)
Mometasone (Nasonex)
Ciclesonide (Zetonna)
Beclomethasone (Beconase, Qnasal)
Triamcinolone (Nasacort AQ)
Budesonide (Rhinocort)
Flunisolide (Nasarel, Nasalide)
Fluticasone propionate (Flonase
Throat lozenges/ cough drops—Cepacol, Major, chloraseptic
Benzocaine, menthol, honey

Table 9

Medications for asthma, COPD

Short-acting anticholinergics:
Ipratropium (Atrovent) two to six puffs q six hours

Long-acting anticholinergics:
Aclidinium Bromide (Tudorza Pressair) one inhalation q twelve hours
Tiotropium (Spiriva) one inhalation/day
Umeclidinium (Incruse, Ellipta) one inhalation/day

Short-acting beta 2 agonists (SABA):
Albuterol inhaler (Ventolin, Accuneb, ProAir, Proventil, Respirol) two puffs q six hours
Levalbuterol (Xopenex) inhaler, two puffs q six hours
Pirbuterol (Maxair) two puffs q six hours
Duoneb (Albuterol/Ipratropium bromide) 3 ml vial inhaled

Long-acting beta agonists:
Arformoterol (Brovana) 2 ml by nebulizer q twelve hours
Salmeterol (Serevent) one cap q twelve hours
Formoterol (Foradil) one cap q twelve hours
Indacaterol (Arcapta) one cap q twenty-four hours

Corticosteroids inhaled:
Beclomethasone (Qvar) two to four puffs q six hours
Budesonide inhalation (Pulmicort) two puffs q twelve hours
Fluticasone propionate (Flovent HFA) two puffs q twelve hours
Fluticasone furoate (Arnuity, Ellipta) one inhalation/day
Mometasone (Asmanex) one to two inhalation q twelve hours

Corticosteroids oral:
Prednisone 5–20 mg PO q twelve hours

Methylxanthines:
Theo-Dur, Slo-Bid 100–200 mg PO q twelve hours (*not used often*)

Leukotriene modifiers:
Montelukast (Singulair) 10 mg PO in a.m.
Zafirlukast (Accolate) 20 mg PO q twelve hours
Zileuton (Zyflo) 600 mg PO q six hours

PDE 4 inhibitor:
Roflumilast (Daliresp) 500 mcg PO/day

Combinations:
Albuterol/Ipratropium (Duoneb, Combivent) two puffs q six hours
Budesonide/Formoterol (Symbicort) two inhalations q twelve hours
Formoterol/ Mometasone (Dulera) one to two inhalations
Salmeterol/Fluticasone- (Advair) one inhalation q twelve hours
Tiotropium/Olodaterol (Stiolto, Respimat) two inhalations q twenty-four hours
Umeclidinium/Vilanterol (Anoro Ellipta) one inhalation q twenty-four hours
Vilanterol/Fluticasone (Breo Ellipta) one inhalation q twenty-four hours
Ephedrine sulfate (Akovaz, Corphedra) for acute bronchospasm 5–10 mg IV
Omalizumab (Xolair) 150–375 mg subQ q two to four weeks

Pulmonary embolism (PE)

A pulmonary artery embolism is an event when a blood clot that forms elsewhere in the body travels to the lungs. Sometimes the clots are small and scattered to the peripheral branches of the pulmonary arteries. At other times, the clots can be massive, occluding the entire lumen of the main pulmonary artery and both branches. Formation of blood clot starts in the venous system of legs or pelvis, which then can migrate into the pulmonary arteries, occluding the lumen of the pulmonary arteries partially or severely, resulting in compromise of oxygen / carbon dioxide exchange, shock, hypotension, and death.

The most frequent causes of PE include hypercoagulation, immobility, trauma, postsurgical state, pelvic fractures, and cancers. Advancing age can be a risk factor. Patients present with sudden onset of dyspnea, pleuritic chest pain, hemoptysis, and hypotension.

V/Q scan shows a mismatch between ventilation and perfusion. D-dimer is usually positive. Chest x-ray shows a nonspecific pattern. Leg ultrasound may show DVT. CT angiogram shows the filling defects in the pulmonary artery.

Prevention includes prophylactic mini anticoagulation with heparin or other anticoagulant agents in patients who are postsurgical or nonambulatory. Sequential compression stockings and pumps are useful. Those who are traveling long distances by airplane, car, or bus are at risk of developing DVT. Recommended guidance includes getting up and moving around periodically and calf exercises, and if necessary, take anticoagulants at prophylactic dosage.

Treatment is immediate anticoagulation with heparin and evaluate for thrombolytic therapy. If the clots are significant and occluding the pulmonary arteries, then catheter-guided administration of TPA into the clot can be lifesaving. Once the patient is stabilized, the anticoagulation is continued for at least six months. If the patient cannot take anticoagulants for whatever reason, then placement of a vena cava filter is recommended as prophylaxis against future events. This procedure can be done percutaneously as a safe technique.

Pneumonia in aging adults

As we age, our body's natural defenses become less dependable, and as a result, older adults are more susceptible to infection, including pneumonia. Potential causes include changes to the respiratory system with age and difficulty in effectively clearing secretions in the bronchial tubes, causing the infection.

Other contributing factors include an aging immune system, which has a harder time fighting off infection, and underlying conditions such as an organ or bone marrow transplant, chemotherapy (treatment for cancer), or long-term steroid use.

Underlying conditions such as diabetes, Parkinson's disease, chemotherapy, and HIV put older adults at a higher risk for pneumonia as well as asthma, COPD (chronic obstructive pulmonary disease), and bronchiectasis. Surgery can also expose older adults to infections that can lead to pneumonia.

Common symptoms include the following:
- Coughing that produces green or yellow fluid such as phlegm
- Lack of energy and confusion
- A sudden spike in fever accompanied by chills
- Abnormally low body temperature
- Severe chest pain
- Shortness of breath / difficulty breathing
- Nausea, vomiting, diarrhea

Diagnostic testing includes a chest x-ray and/or CBC and a procalcitonin test. Sometimes a chest CT can delineate pneumonia that might have eluded detection with CXR. Bacterial pneumonia is usually treated with antibiotics. If the infection is viral, an antiviral medicine may be prescribed. Besides medication, IV fluids, oxygen, pain relief and medical support are provided.

Options to help reduce the risk of pneumonia include the following:
- Get vaccinated. All people over age sixty-five should get an annual flu shot as well as a pneumococcal vaccine and Prevnar—a onetime shot that protects against the pneumococcus, or pneumonia bacteria.
- Practice good hygiene. Wash your hands regularly or use an alcohol-based hand sanitizer.
- Do not smoke or take steps to quit. Smoking negatively affects the lungs. Those who smoke are at a greater overall risk of pneumonia because the lungs' defense mechanisms become compromised.
- Practice a healthy lifestyle. Follow a healthy diet and exercise regimen. These actions will help bolster the immune system and reduce the risk of pneumonia.

Bronchiectasis

Bronchiectasis is an uncommon disease, most often secondary to an infectious process, which results in the abnormal and permanent distortion of one or more of the conducting bronchi airway passages.

Clinical manifestations of bronchiectasis are the following:
- Cough and daily mucopurulent sputum production, often lasting months to years
- Blood-streaked sputum or hemoptysis from airway damage associated with acute infection
- Dyspnea, pleuritic chest pain, wheezing, fever, weakness, fatigue, and weight loss
- (Rarely) episodic hemoptysis with little to no sputum production (i.e., dry bronchiectasis)

Exacerbations of bronchiectasis from acute bacterial infections may produce the following signs:
- Increased sputum production over baseline
- Increased viscosity of sputum
- A foul odor of the sputum
- Low-grade fever
- Increased constitutional symptoms (fatigue, malaise)
- Increased dyspnea, shortness of breath, wheezing, or pleuritic pain

The diagnosis of bronchiectasis involves the following:
- A compatible history of chronic respiratory symptoms (e.g., daily cough and purulent sputum production)
- Sputum analysis, which may strengthen clinical suspicion
- Chest radiography, which is occasionally sufficient for confirming the diagnosis
- High-resolution computed tomography (HRCT) scanning, which is the standard test for diagnosis

Treatment modalities include the following:
- Antibiotics and chest physiotherapy
- Bronchodilators
- Corticosteroid therapy
- Dietary supplementation
- Oxygen (for hypoxemic patients with severe disease)
- Hospitalization for severe exacerbations
- Surgical therapies in selected situations

Acceptable antibiotic regimens for mild to moderately ill outpatients include seven to ten days of the following:

- Amoxicillin
- Tetracycline
- Trimethoprim-sulfamethoxazole
- Macrolide (azithromycin or clarithromycin)
- Second-generation cephalosporins
- Fluoroquinolones

Chapter 7

Cancer

Advancing age increases susceptibility to getting cancer. It is unclear as to why older adults are more likely to get cancer than younger adults. Their mutations go unchecked and unregulated in the older individuals. Cancers of the oral cavity, GI tract, liver, pancreas, skin and soft tissues, lungs and breasts, thyroid, and prostate, uterine, and ovarian origin are all more common in the older adult as compared to young adults. Cancers do behave differently in the younger population versus the older adult.

Lung cancer

Smoking is considered the major causative factor. Lung cancer is the most common among cancers that result in death of older adults. Patients present with symptoms of chronic cough, hemoptysis, dyspnea, and enlarged lymph nodes in the neck. Lung cancer is often detected as an incidental finding on chest x-rays or CT scan of the chest done for some other reason. The diagnosis is confirmed with thin cut CT scans, bronchoscopy, mediastinoscopy, percutaneous CT-guided biopsy, and finally at surgery.

Staging of the disease and biology of the tumor are deciding factors on treatment options.

For non-small cell cancers that include adenocarcinoma and squamous cell carcinoma, surgery is the first line of treatment. This may involve lobectomy or pneumonectomy. Radiation and/or chemotherapy may follow this, depending upon the staging. For small cell lung cancers, radiation and chemotherapy are the first line of treatment.

Breast cancer

Breast cancer is the most common cancer among women. Women above age fifty are at highest risk and are more likely to have well-differentiated adenocarcinoma. Late menarche and menopause, nulliparity, smoking, lack of exercise, previous breast disorders, and hormone medications are risk factors. Patients may present with a palpable mass. Often, they are discovered upon a routine screening mammogram as a nonpalpable abnormality such as microcalcification or soft tissue density. The best screening test is still mammography. However, there is debate about the value of doing routine screening mammograms in older adults. The American Geriatric Society recommends screening mammograms on asymptomatic patients up to the age of eighty-five. Other organizations limit it up to the age of seventy-five. Fine needle aspiration cytology under sonogram guidance or a core needle biopsy under stereotactic mammotome procedure is often done for histological diagnosis and for hormone assay studies. Open surgical biopsy is a less desired option to confirm a diagnosis.

Surgery is the mainstay of treatment, which hopes to remove the entire cancer bearing area. This can be accomplished with a wide excision lumpectomy or modified radical mastectomy. Spread to regional lymphatics is assessed by doing sentinel lymph node biopsy. If the sentinel node is positive for metastasis, full axillary lymph node dissection is the next step in the evaluation. Whenever possible, breast conservation and limited axillary node dissections are offered to the patient. There are cases where one would be better off doing a modified radical mastectomy. Older women may prefer a modified radical mastectomy over conservative surgery since they may not want to go through a prolonged course of radiation therapy, hormone therapy, or chemotherapy and would not be overly concerned about cosmetic appearance. Radiation therapy, chemotherapy, or hormone therapy follow surgery. Choices for therapy depend on the stage of disease, presence of metastasis, and hormone assay results. With early detection and treatment of breast cancer, an 80 to 90 percent cure rate is expected. In the very older adult and debilitated patients there is room to treat breast cancer by conservative surgery to remove the cancer mass alone and not provide the full spectrum of adjuvant therapy.

Colorectal cancers

Colorectal cancer is the third leading cancer among older adults after lung and breast. The incidence is highest after age sixty-five. Most common predisposing condition is adenomatous polyp. The mucosa can undergo areas of neoplastic transformation for unknown reasons. Ulcerative colitis, Crohn's colitis, and familial polyposis are other risk factors. Diets made up of animal hydrocarbons are considered as higher risk when compared to a vegetarian and bulky diet. Patients complain of abdominal discomfort, alteration of bowel habits, bleeding per rectum, and abdominal distension due to obstruction. Stool for occult blood is the first line of screening. Other fecal analyses are Cologuard test and fecal immunoassay test (FIT test). Patients may be anemic with iron deficiency. Colonoscopy is the most definitive diagnostic procedure during which biopsies can be obtained and polyps can be excised. Definitive treatment is by surgical removal of the affected part of the GI tract. This may be in the form of right hemicolectomy, resection of segments of transverse colon, left hemicolectomy, or sigmoid colon resection or abdominoperineal resection. Whenever possible, the bowel ends are reanastomosed. Otherwise, a colostomy is done. Following surgery, depending upon the stage of the disease, adjuvant therapy in the form of radiation or chemotherapy is recommended. Common locations for metastasis are the liver. If there is a solitary metastasis, partial hepatectomy followed by adjuvant chemotherapy can prolong life. If colon cancer is left untreated, it leads to obstruction, bleeding, perforation, and metastasis. Emergency surgery leads to more complications and incurability compared to elective early surgery.

Prostate cancer

Prostate cancer affects the older adult male frequently. Ninety-five percent are adenocarcinoma. The remaining are squamous or transitional cell cancers. Older age increases the prevalence. Black men are at higher risk. There is a familial incidence, and it is related to hormones. Prostate specific antigen (PSA) is a good screening test but not specific. However, progressively rising levels of PSA or elevated levels of PSA are indicative of higher risk for prostate cancer. Controversy remains about routine screening with PSA levels since it can lead to over detection and unnecessary treatments. Sonogram and ultrasound-guided needle biopsy are diagnostic. Initially, prostate cancer can be asymptomatic. As it advances, there can be symptoms of hematuria, hematospermia, urgency, frequency, and hesitancy. Rarely the first symptom could be bone pain from metastatic bone deposits. Rectal examination reveals one or more nodules, induration, or asymmetry. Spread of disease occurs via bloodstream to bones, which gives a denser bone tissue pattern or to brain, lungs, and distant organs. Spread can also be to regional lymph nodes in pelvis and para-aortic region. Treatment is controversial since most patients do not die from prostate cancer itself but from other illnesses. Treatment options include radical prostatectomy by use of robotics to do nerve-sparing surgery or by open method or radiation therapy or androgen suppression therapy by orchiectomy or by medications.

Most patients prefer to have surgery done for early cancers. Advanced cancers are best treated by palliative care. If a person has a life expectancy of less than five years, prostate cancer can be left untreated.

Ovarian cancer

Ovarian cancer is one of the common cancers in older women. Two-thirds occur in post-menopausal women. It is a silent killer since it can grow to an advanced level with very few symptoms. Initial symptoms are vague with lower abdominal discomfort, nausea, dyspepsia, and urinary frequency. The tumor can grow slowly to an exceptionally enormous size and can expand into the abdominal cavity with little pressure on neighboring organs. The first presenting symptom could be a distended abdomen with ascites. Tumor markers of CA-125 and CEA are helpful but not specific. Ultrasound of the abdomen and CT scan are diagnostic. A surgical debulking procedure is performed in all cases even if it is advanced since postoperative chemotherapy can be effective. Surgery involves total salpingo-oophorectomy and total hysterectomy along with maximal debulking of the metastatic disease. This may involve omentectomy and para-aortic and iliac lymphadenectomy. Life expectancy can be extended by years with aggressive therapy.

Cervical cancer

Cervical cancer was once the leading cause of cancer in Western society, but it is no longer. Pap smears became a part of regular checkups or gynecological exams, making it possible to detect the disease early, preventing it from becoming fatal.

The rate of death for women over the age of sixty-five from cervical cancer is higher than that of women below that age, and 25 percent of new cases occur among older adults. Of that group of older women, approximately 7.6 per 100,000 die from cervical cancer, as compared to only 2.1 for younger women.

Studies show that so many older women die simply because they choose to not have Pap smears, putting them in jeopardy.

In younger women and with the advent of the HPV vaccination, now have a reduced risk. Women have been told that they do not have to get a Pap test for cervical cancer if they are over the age of sixty-five, but according to researchers, the data does not support that recommendation.

Health-care professionals are encouraged to discuss the inclusion of Pap smears for aging women at least every three years.

The primary symptom of cervical cancer is abnormal bleeding or vaginal discharge, which can also be symptomatic of cancers of the ovaries or uterus. If a woman experiences these symptoms, it is important to seek medical attention as soon as possible and not wait until an annual exam. Other symptoms can include fatigue, nausea, or weight loss.

Treatment options for older patients with cervical cancer are limited, as often the patient presents with it at an advanced stage. Treatment of localized cervical cancer includes surgery, brachytherapy, and concomitant radio- and chemotherapy. However, the risk-benefit balance for these treatments among older patients has been poorly studied. Treatment decisions in older patients are complex due to frequent comorbidities and age-related impairments such as malnutrition, functional dependence, cognitive decline, and sensitivity to treatment toxicity. Therefore, the treatment of cervical carcinoma is not consistent in the geriatric population.

Uterine cancer

Endometrial cancer is the most common gynecologic cancer, and with a median age of sixty-two at diagnosis, it affects a substantial number of older women. With increasing age and obesity rates in the world's population, a concomitant increase in older women with endometrial cancer is predicted. Older women are more likely to die of endometrial cancer compared to younger patients. The reasons for the higher mortality rate include more aggressive tumor biology, less favorable clinicopathologic features, and more advanced disease. Other factors are reluctance to offer surgical treatment to older patients and complications of treatment. The management of endometrial cancer requires a multidisciplinary approach (surgery, radiation therapy, and systemic chemotherapy). For each one of these treatment options, the feasibility (related to the technical aspects of the procedure/treatment), side effects, safety (related to older-patient factors), and the overall benefit as it pertains to older women with endometrial cancer should be assessed carefully.

Chapter 8

Diabetes Mellitus

Diabetes mellitus (DM) is a metabolic disorder resulting from impaired insulin secretion or insulin action resulting in hyperglycemia and a series of systemic effects as a sequel. Twenty percent of the adult population has diabetes mellitus. There is impaired and delayed release of insulin as well as increased resistance to insulin with advancing age. Glucotoxicity leads to a variety of metabolic complications with multiple organ dysfunction and decreased life expectancy.

Type 1 is the early onset or juvenile diabetes due to lack of insulin production. It is an autoimmune disorder where insulin-producing beta cells in the pancreas are destroyed. Type 2 is adult-onset diabetes due to insulin resistance or lack of compensatory insulin response, which progressively gets worse with advancing age. The pancreatic beta cells are unable to keep up with the need for insulin.

The first symptoms are polyuria, polyphagia, and polydipsia, and they may be accompanied by unexplained weight loss. Varying negative consequences of uncontrolled diabetes mellitus occur.

Aftereffects of uncontrolled diabetes mellitus include increased chance for cardiovascular disorders, hypertension, angina, myocardial infarction, nephropathy, retinopathy, skin infections, soft tissue infections, obesity, ketoacidosis, hyperlipidemia, neurological disorders, neuropathy, Charcot's joints, peripheral gangrene, micro aneurysms, autonomic neuropathy leading to gastroparesis, postural hypotension, atonic bladder, cognitive disorders, depression, and entrapment syndromes such as carpal tunnel syndrome.

Acute complications are diabetic ketoacidosis (DKA), hypoglycemic episodes, and acute infections. In DKA, there is hyperglycemia with hyperosmolar state, acidosis, free fatty acid metabolism, and lipolysis due to decreased glucose metabolism. Patients exhibits dehydration, dyspnea, abdominal pain, vomiting, altered mentation and coma, oliguria, and renal failure. Precipitating factors can be acute infections, pneumonia, myocardial infarction, or stroke. Treatment includes rapid rehydration, correction of hyperglycemia with insulin, correction of initiating causes, and other supportive measures.

The diagnosis of diabetes is arrived at from a fasting blood sugar above 126 mg/dl. Physicians rely on HbA1c of above 6 as highly suggestive of the diagnosis as well.

Treatment includes diet, exercise, weight loss programs, and medications. Various caloric or carbohydrate restricted diabetic diets help control blood glucose levels. They aim to reduce sugars, carbohydrates, trans fats, cholesterol, and calorie counts. Moderate activity or exercise for 150 minutes per week is the minimum requirement. Medications are oral or injectable. Medications are listed in the table that follows. Glycemic control in older adults need not be below 6.0. Such tight control may lead to hypoglycemia complications; hence Hb A1c of 7.0 is acceptable.

It is important to avoid hypoglycemia while the patient is on insulin or other medications. Evaluation for comorbid conditions and complications of diabetes mellitus are included in the workup in all cases. Older patients with diabetes can develop cognitive impairment, depression, urinary incontinence, falls and fractures, and functional limitations.

For decades, metformin served as the foundation for type 2 diabetes treatment. However, the landscape has shifted dramatically in recent years with the introduction of Glucagon-like Peptide-1 (GLP-1) receptor agonists.

The story begins in 2005 with the FDA approval of the first GLP-1 agonist for type 2 diabetes. These medications mimic a natural gut hormone that stimulates insulin release and lowers blood sugar levels. This translates to a more potent and sustained approach to blood sugar control compared to traditional medications, helping a sizable portion of patients achieve glycemic targets (HbA1c).

A landmark development came in 2017 with the introduction of Ozempic (semaglutide). This medication, along with others in the GLP-1 agonist class like Dulaglutide (Trulicity) and Tirzepatide (Mounjaro), offer added benefits beyond blood sugar control. They have been shown to promote weight loss, a crucial factor in managing type 2 diabetes. Recent studies also suggest potential reductions in cardiovascular events and anti-inflammatory effects (see Chapter 21 for further details on obesity management).

Despite these advancements, challenges remain. Supply chain issues can limit access to some GLP-1 medications, and the injectable nature may not be suitable for all patients. Additionally, the cost can be a significant obstacle.

In conclusion, GLP-1 receptor agonists represent a major leap forward in type 2 diabetes management, offering improved blood sugar control, weight management benefits, and potential cardiovascular advantages. However, ensuring access and affordability remains an ongoing challenge.

Table 10

Medications for treatment of diabetes mellitus

Oral noninsulin agents

Biguanide: decreases hepatic glucose production
Metformin (Glucophage, Glumetza, Fortamet) 500–2,550 mg in divided doses

Second-generation sulfonylureas: increases insulin secretion
Glimepiride (Amaryl) 4–8 mg once daily
Glipizide (Glucotrol) 2.5–40 mg in divided doses or once daily
Glyburide (Micronase, Glynase) 1.25–20 mg in divided doses or once daily

Alpha-glucosidase inhibitors: delays glucose absorption
Acarbose (Precose) 50–100 mg q eight hours
Miglitol (Glyset) 25–100 mg q eight hours

DPP-4 enzyme inhibitors: protects and enhances endogenous incretin hormones (Incretins are gut peptide metabolic hormones released after eating, which encourages the pancreatic islet cells to release insulin, thus reducing blood sugar.)
Alogliptin (Nesina) 25 mg once a day
Linagliptin (Tradjenta) 5 mg once a day
Sitagliptin (Januvia) 50–100 mg once daily
Saxagliptin (Onglyza) 2.5–5 mg once daily

Meglitinides: increases insulin secretion
Nateglinide (Starlix) 60–120 mg before meals
Repaglinide (Prandin) 0.5–4 mg before meals

Thiazolidinedione: insulin resistance reducers
Pioglitazone (Actos) 15–45 mg per day
Rosiglitazone (Avandia) 4 mg q twelve to twenty-four hours

SGLT2 inhibitors decreases glucose reabsorption from kidneys
Canagliflozin (Invokana) 100–300 mg per day
Dapagliflozin (Farxiga) 5–10 mg per day
Empagliflozin (Jardiance) 10–25 mg per day

Others
Bromocriptine (Cycloset) 1.6–4.8 mg per day
Colesevelam (Welchol) 3,750 mg per day

Combinations
Glipizide and Metformin (Metaglip) 2.5/250 mg per day
Glyburide and Metformin (Glucovance) 2.5/500 mg per day
Pioglitazone and metformin (Actoplus met) 15/850 mg q
twelve to twenty-four hours
Repaglinide and metformin (PrandiMet) 1/500–4/1,000 q
twelve hours
Rosiglitazone and metformin (Avandamet) 2/500 q twelve hours
Rosiglitazone and glimepiride (Avandaryl) 4/1 mg per day
Pioglitazone and glimepiride (Duetact) 30/2 mg per day
Saxagliptin and metformin (Kombiglyze XR) 5/1,000 per day
Sitagliptin and metformin (Janumet) 100/2,000 mg in divided doses
Linagliptin and metformin (Jentadueto) 2.5 mg/1,000 mg
two tabs once a day
Alogliptin and metformin (Kazano) 12 mg/500 mg
Alogliptin and pioglitazone (Oseni) 25/15 to 25/45 mg daily
Empaglifozin/linagliptin (Glyxambi) 10/5 to 25/5 daily
Canagliflozin/metformin (Invokamet) 50/500 to 150/1,000,
one to two tabs twice a day

Injectable noninsulin agents
GLP 1 receptor agonists:
Dulaglutide (Trulicity) 0.75–1.5 mg SubQ once a week
Exenatide (Byetta) 5–10 mcg SubQ twice daily
Exenatide extended release (Bydureon) 2 mg SubQ once a week
Liraglutide (Victoza) 0.6–1.8 mg SubQ once a day
Semaglutide (Ozempic, Wegovy,) 0.25 mg, 0.5 mg, 1 mg weekly
Tirzepatide (Monjorouo) 2.5mg, 5mg, 10mg, 12.5mg, 15 mg wkly

Amylin analog
Pramlintide (Symlin) 60–120 mcg SubQ before meals
Insulin preparations
Rapid acting: onset fifteen to twenty minutes, peak
0.5–1.5 hours, duration three to four hours
Insulin glulisine (Apidra) 1 ml–100 units Sub
Insulin lispro (Humalog) 0.5–1 unit/kg/day (100 units/ml) SubQ
Insulin aspart (Novolog)—same
Inhaled (Afrezza) four units inhaled same as four units SubQ

Regular acting: Onset 0.5–1 hour, peak two to three hours,
duration five to eight hours
Humulin 100 units/ml, 0.5 units/kg/day SubQ
Novolin—same

Long or intermediate acting: onset 1–1.5 hour, peak four to twelve
hours, duration twenty-four hours
NPH (Humulin, Novolin)—same
Insulin detemir (Levemir)—same
Insulin glargine (Lantus, Toujeo) 0.2–0.5 units/kg/day

Combinations: peak two to twelve hours, duration
twenty-four hours
Isophane insulin and regular insulin (Novolin 70/30)
Insulin lispro protamine and insulin lispro (Humalog mix 50/50 or
75/25)

Chapter 9

Endocrine Disorders

Thyroid

Thyroid disease. As adults age, they become more susceptible to thyroid disease, which affects the body's metabolic rate. Early detection and proper treatment can limit the effects of the conditions and ensure that older adults continue to live healthy lives. About 20 percent of women over the age of sixty have some form of thyroid disease.

Hypothyroidism is more common in older adults, but it is a challenge to recognize it because symptoms occur over many years. Aging adults with this disease may have only one or two symptoms. The presentation of symptoms depends on the deficiency of the thyroid hormones T4 and T3.

Symptoms of hypothyroidism vary depending on how low the thyroid hormone levels are, and may include fatigue; sluggishness; an increased sensitivity to cold; constipation; pale, dry skin; a puffy face; hoarseness; high cholesterol levels; brittle hair and nails; unexplained weight gain; muscle aches; tenderness and stiffness; menstrual changes; muscle weakness; pain; stiffness or swelling in the joints; and depression.

Risk factors for developing hypothyroidism include females over the age of fifty, a family history of autoimmune diseases, previous radiation treatment in the upper neck and/or chest area, prior surgery on the thyroid gland, and iodine deficiency. Treatment is the replacement of the deficient hormone with a synthetic thyroid hormone.

Hyperthyroidism presents itself in many ways, making it a challenge to diagnose as its symptoms are indicative of other health conditions. Adults may present only one or two symptoms of this disease. Medications can cause the same symptoms or even mask the signs of this disease.

Symptoms of hyperthyroidism may include sudden weight loss; rapid or irregular heartbeat; pounding of the heart; increased appetite; nervousness, anxiety, or irritability; tremors in the hands and/or fingers; sweating; menstrual changes; an increased sensitivity to heat; changes in bowel patterns; an enlarged thyroid gland; fatigue; muscle weakness; and difficulty sleeping.

Risk factors for developing hyperthyroidism include a family history of hyperthyroidism, prior history of Graves' or Plummer's disease, thyroiditis, or a toxic adenoma on the thyroid gland.

Thyroid disease can be more difficult to diagnose in aging adults. When diagnosed and properly treated, thyroid disease can be managed, and quality of life improves. Antithyroid medications commonly used as initial treatment or for long-term use include methimazole, carbimazole, and propylthiouracil.

Options for the long-term treatment of hyperthyroidism include medical management with antithyroid medications or thyroid ablative therapy in the form of surgery or radioiodine therapy. Radioiodine is preferred over surgery in the elderly with hyperthyroidism because of the increased morbidity and mortality associated with surgery.

Thyroid nodules and cancer. The prevalence of thyroid nodules increases with age. Ultrasound studies reveal a 40–60 percent prevalence of thyroid nodules in the elderly population. Clinically significant thyroid nodules are also more prevalent in the aging population. Fortunately, malignancy is present in only 10 percent of the nodules, and the frequency is similar or lower in younger patients with thyroid nodules. Ruling out a malignancy in thyroid nodules is important to avoid unnecessary investigations in over 90 percent of the benign lesions. Fine needle aspiration biopsy revolutionized the diagnosis of thyroid nodules, and the diagnostic accuracy depends on the person performing the procedure and the cytopathologist. Ultrasound-guided aspiration has improved the diagnostic accuracy of fine needle aspiration biopsy. Malignant lesions need surgery, and benign lesions need yearly follow-up. Indeterminate or suspicious lesions in FNAC require excision biopsy, and up to 15 percent of these suspicious lesions prove to be malignant at the time of surgery.

Amiodarone-induced thyrotoxicosis. Amiodarone-induced thyrotoxicosis (AIT) requires special attention in aging cardiac patients as amiodarone is one of the first-line drugs used in atrial fibrillation. Amiodarone causes two types of thyroid disease: one with preexisting multinodular goiter and the other with destructive thyroiditis. Although both types are self-limiting, sometimes severe forms of disease can occur that may require high doses of glucocorticoids, antithyroid medications, and sometimes surgery. Discontinuation of amiodarone will not immediately improve the condition due to the prolonged half-life of the drug, and discontinuation may not be feasible because of underlying cardiac disease.

Parathyroid disease. Primary hyperparathyroidism (PHPT) is more frequent than hypoparathyroidism, and its prevalence increases with age. Clinical presentations mimic normal aging. Diagnosis is often incidental and detected by mild hypercalcemia. Serum PTH may present diagnostic uncertainties in the elderly due to the lack of standardized values by age groups. Both the progression of hypercalcemia and the systemic involvement of PHPT appear to be lower in older patients as compared to younger ones. Parathyroidectomy is the treatment of choice in all patients with hyperparathyroidism regardless of age to reduce the fracture risk. Ultrasound and scintigraphy with 99mTc sestamibi allow the performing of a minimally invasive parathyroidectomy in most patients. A cure rate for older patients after a parathyroidectomy is of over 95 percent with extremely low rates of complications and no mortality.

Hypoparathyroidism in older patients is uncommon and mostly secondary to neck surgery. Neuromuscular and psychiatric manifestations of hypocalcemia are predominant. In the presence of hypocalcemia, the diagnosis is based on an inappropriately low PTH. The treatment of chronic hypocalcemia is Ca and calcitriol. The goal of therapy is to avoid hypocalcemia, hyperphosphatemia, and hypercalciuria.

Chapter 10

Kidney Disorders

Chronic renal failure and the need for dialysis are of great concern for aging patients. With advancing age, there is a natural reduction in the glomerular filtration rate. Symptoms may not be apparent until the disease progresses. Symptoms include sleep disturbances, increased body weight, nausea and vomiting, dyspnea, fatigue, lower-extremity edema, muscle cramps, peripheral neuropathy, and neurological disorders.

Slow and progressive dysfunction of the kidneys can be due to type 2 diabetes mellitus, vascular disorders, hypertension, medication effects, cancer conditions, prostate problems, exposure to allergens such as contrast dye, chronic glomerulonephritis, or hereditary conditions.

Initially, there is increased excretion of albumin in the urine. Glomerular filtration rate goes down, and there is a slow but steady rise in blood urea nitrogen and creatinine levels. Hyperkalemia and acidosis occur. Creatinine levels above 10 and potassium above 6 mg/L can cause cardiac arrest.

Diagnosis is by urinalysis and blood chemistry profiles. Subsequently, a renal ultrasound is performed to evaluate obstructive pathology, stones, and tumors. A MR angiogram or CT angiogram can assess renal artery stenosis. In selected cases, a renal biopsy may be necessary.

In the early stage, medical treatment is started by controlling blood pressure using ACE inhibitors, controlling diabetes mellitus, dietary restriction of proteins, treating hyperlipidemia and avoiding triamterene, and NSAIDs. Other measures are to reduce dietary potassium, increase calcium intake and treat vitamin D insufficiency and anemia.

In the advanced cases, one should plan for dialysis rather than facing an avoidable crisis and emergency dialysis. Discussion with the patient and family about options of hemodialysis and peritoneal dialysis is entertained. An arteriovenous fistula is created, allowing it to mature for eight weeks before use for dialysis. Autogenous AV fistulas are far superior to AV grafts made of synthetic materials. An alternative to dialysis is renal transplantation for younger patients.

Chronic renal failure in older adult patients carries a poor prognosis. Multiple medical comorbidities and dialysis-related complications tether the patient to the hospital with repeated admissions.

The survival in the geriatric population is anywhere from five months to thirty-six months. Initial benefits of dialysis become a burden over time, and patients may decide to withdraw from further care to accept hospice or palliative care.

Acute renal failure or acute tubular necrosis can occur in situations of shock, sepsis, or anaphylactic reactions. Common scenarios are hypovolemic shock following severe dehydration, blood loss, trauma, or burns. Third spacing can occur in cases of severe sepsis or acute pancreatitis. Medications such as aminoglycosides, radiology contrast materials, and other drugs can precipitate acute renal shutdown. Other causes are multiple myeloma or thromboembolic events.

In the early stage, as it is evolving, one should try to correct the underlying problem as best as possible. Hydration and a fluid challenge are done in all shock states. Blood pressure is supported with low doses of dopamine to maintain renal blood flow. Monitoring is performed with a central line or Swan-Ganz catheter to ensure adequate preload. Blood loss is replaced with blood or plasma. Potential allergens are stopped, and treatment is initiated with steroids. If these are of no avail, then increasing doses of diuretics can be instituted, hoping to improve renal output. In the meantime, metabolic corrections are done to keep potassium, calcium, phosphorus, and magnesium at optimal levels. Anemia is corrected, and blood volume is maintained at optimal levels.

Once it is confirmed that acute renal failure has developed, it is best to watch patiently for potential reversal. One may need to perform one or two sessions of temporary hemodialysis. Indications for emergency dialysis would be hyperkalemia, acidosis, and volume overload. Many times, after a week or two, a recovery can occur. Patients may go into a diuretic phase and need monitoring for a hypovolemic state.

Strict intake and output measurements and monitoring of daily weights, daily electrolytes, nutritional needs, infection control and cardiopulmonary assessments are done.

Table 11

Medication list of diuretics

Loop-acting diuretics:
Bumex 0.5–2 mg PO
Demadex 10–20 mg PO
Edecrin 50–100 mg PO
Lasix 40 mg PO or IV

Potassium-sparing diuretics:
Aldactone 25–100 mg PO
Dyrenium 100 mg PO
Midamor 5 mg PO

Thiazides:
Hydrochlorothiazide 12.5–50 mg daily
Chlorthalidone 12.5–50 mg daily
Metolazone 2.5–20 mg daily

Chapter 11

Urological Disorders

Urological problems are common for both men and women as they age. Men are afflicted with prostate enlargement, prostate cancer, and scrotal and penile problems. Women have problems with recurrent urinary tract infections, stress incontinence, prolapse of uterus, and vaginal infections. Both sexes are at risk for sexually transmitted disorders, renal stones, and cancers.

Benign hypertrophy of prostate (BPH)

By far, BPH is the most common urological problem affecting older adult male patients. An enlarged prostate gland obstructs the prostatic urethra, causing dysuria, hesitancy, frequency, urgency, nocturia, hematuria, weak urinary stream, and retention of urine. Uncorrected, there could be obstruction and back pressure into the ureters resulting in hydronephrosis or complete retention of urine, needing emergency intervention such as catheterization or suprapubic cystostomy.

Physical examination reveals an enlarged prostate on rectal examination with smooth bilobular mass projecting into the rectal canal. Postvoiding residual urine is increased to 100 ml or more. Sonography done transrectally and transabdominally shows the enlargement of the prostate. Urinalysis shows occasional white blood cells or red blood cells. Blood chemistry defines renal function.

Medical therapy is helpful for most patients. Tamsulosin (Flomax), silodosin (Rapaflo), or alfuzosin (Uroxatral) is the first line of therapy. The second line of medications are finasteride (Proscar) or dutasteride (Avodart). They can cause erectile dysfunction and gynaecomastia.

If medical therapy fails or if the patient chooses, surgery is the next option. Transurethral resection of the prostate is still the best choice. Recently new methods have been developed which include laser therapy, microwave therapy, and open prostatectomy.

Table 12

Medications for benign hypertrophy of prostate

Alpha-1 blockers—relaxes prostate and bladder detrusor smooth muscle

First generation:
Terazosin (Hytrin) 1–10 mg per day
Doxazosin (Cardura) 0.5–16 mg per day

Second generation:
Tamsulosin (Flomax) 0.4–0.8 mg per day
Silodosin (Rapaflo) 4–8 mg per day
5 alpha reductase inhibitors: reduces prostate size
Finasteride (Proscar, Propecia) 5 mg per day
Dutasteride (Avodart) 0.5 mg per day

Cancer of prostate

Prostate cancer is slow growing and causes the same symptoms as benign hypertrophy of the prostate as described above. Physical examination reveals a palpable nodule on the prostate by rectal examination. Sonography shows nodules in the prostate, and FNA under ultrasound guidance confirms the malignancy. Prostate-specific antigen (PSA) is a tumor marker blood test. An elevated PSA should lead to suspicion of prostate cancer. Follow-up repeat blood tests of PSA is useful to know the state of the disease.

Prostate cancer is disseminated via the bloodstream to the spine and other long bones. The images show up as denser areas on plain x-ray since the metastasis is osteoblastic as compared to osteolytic for other bony metastases. Bone scan, MR scan, or PET scan can confirm metastatic disease as well. A considerable number of patients can live long lives even with metastatic disease.

Treatment is by surgery, radiotherapy, hormone therapy, or just palliative therapy.

Surgery can be radical prostatectomy by open method or by robotic assisted method. Radiotherapy is by radon seed implants into the prostate gland. Those who are suitable for surgery have the benefit of cure with no further follow-up therapy. Robotic assisted radical prostatectomy offers a minimally invasive procedure with a low rate of incontinence and preservation of sexual function. A disadvantage of radiotherapy is cystitis and bladder contracture over a period of years.

Once prostate cancer has advanced, some urologists and oncologists will recommend only clinical follow-up and symptomatic palliative care since treatment does not increase life expectancy. Hormone therapies such as orchiectomy or antitestosterone medications are also recommended.

Table 13

Medications for prostate cancer

GnRH agonists:
Goserelin acetate (Zoladex) 3.6 mg SubQ once a month
Leuprolide acetate (Lupron Depot) 7.5 mg SubQ once a month
Triptorelin (Trelstar Depot) 3.75 mg IM once a month
Histrelin acetate (Vantas) 50 mg subQ implant once a year

Antiandrogens:
Bicalutamide (Casodex) 50 mg daily
Flutamide (Eulexin) 250 mg po q eight hours
Nilutamide (Nilandron) 300 mg PO daily times thirty days
GnRH antagonist
Degarelix (Firmagon) 240 mg subQ, then 80 mg subQ once a month

---

Urinary incontinence

Urinary incontinence is involuntary leakage of urine, causing hygienic and personal care problems. It is a source of social embarrassment and often goes unreported. It is a health-care problem involving perineal care, hygienic concerns, skin infections, and decubitus care. Micturition is a function of urologic, neurologic, muscular, and cognitive control. Incontinence can be due to functional problems, stress incontinence, or overflow incontinence. With advancing age, incontinence can be due to multifactorial issues such as neurological deficits, psychological problems, dementia, loss of sphincter control, overflow secondary to retention, prolapse of pelvic floor and functional impairment, fecal impaction, medication effects, or spinal cord problems. In others, it is due to irritation of the bladder secondary to infections, stones, or tumors. Stress incontinence is leakage when there is increased intra-abdominal pressure such as coughing, laughing, or straining. The sphincter has weakened due to trauma related to childbirth or injuries or pelvic floor weakness. Another cause is due to contracted bladder from radiation effects or chronic cystitis.

The workup of the patient includes urodynamic studies, ultrasound of bladder, kidneys, and residual bladder contents after complete micturition, urinalysis, blood tests, urinary stress test, and cystoscopy.

The treatment for incontinence is based on the cause. Perineal care with suitable diapers or moisture-absorbing garments can be provided, and the older individuals may need added nursing care. Prevention of skin damage, ulcerations, or decubitus ulcers is essential. Surgery to correct pelvic floor prolapse and sphincter procedures and to correct obstructive pathologies such as enlarged prostate are considered. Pelvic muscle training, scheduled/timed voiding, and habit training are recommended. Medications can be effective as itemized in the following table.

Table 14

Medications used in treatment of urinary incontinence

Estrogens:
Estradiol vaginal tablets 10–25 mcg
Estradiol ring 2 mg ring once every ninety days
Estrogen vaginal cream 0.5–2 mg

Antimuscarinics:
Darifenacin (Enablex) 7.5–15 mg daily
Fesoterodine (Toviaz) 4–8 mg daily
Oxybutynin (Ditropan) 2.5–5 mg twice daily
Solifenacin (Vesicare) 5–10 mg daily

Tolterodine (Detrol) 1–2 mg twice daily
Trospium (Sanctura) 20 mg twice daily

Alpha-1 adrenergic blockers:
Prazosin 1–10 mg three times daily
Doxazosin 1–8 mg daily
Terazosin 1–20 mg daily
Alfuzosin 10 mg daily
Silodosin 8 mg daily
Tamsulosin 0.4–0.8 mg daily

5 alpha reductase inhibitors:
Finasteride 5 mg daily
Dutasteride 0.5 mg daily

Others:
Bethanechol 10–50 mg three times daily
Desmopressin 0.2–0.6 mg daily
Imipramine 25 mg three times daily

Urinary tract infections (UTI)

Recurrent catheterizations or instrumentations or indwelling catheters are well-established contributors to acute UTIs. Women are more susceptible to urinary tract infections and have higher incidences of cystitis and pyelonephritis. UTI symptoms include urgency, frequency and hesitancy. Urine can be discolored and foul smelling. Urinalysis reveals red and white blood cells. Urine cultures usually show E. coli. Other offending bacteria are Proteus mirabilis, Klebsiella, Enterobacter, Serratia, and Pseudomonas aeruginosa. Underlying factors could be stones, tumors, benign hypertrophy of the prostate, honeymoon cystitis, change in hormone status of the older adult, fecal incontinence, diabetes mellitus, stroke, neurological disorders, weakened pelvic floor, or radiation.

Severe urinary tract infections can cause fever, chills, frequency, hematuria, dysuria, and abdominal or flank pain. There may be suprapubic tenderness or renal angle tenderness. Many UTIs require hospitalization for intravenous antibiotics and hydration. Milder forms can be treated with oral antibiotics and hydration.

Chapter 12

Neurological Disorders

Dementia is a progressive decline in cognitive functions sufficient to affect daily functions. The cause of the dementing illness can be due to Alzheimer's disease, Lewy body dementia, vascular dementia, or frontotemporal dementia. Patients may have memory loss, language problems, learning difficulties, visual disturbances, indifference, agitation, personality changes, or hallucinations. The onset is slow, and initial symptoms are considered age-related problems, thus getting medical attention only in later stages. By this time memory loss becomes obvious. Disorientation of time and place occurs, eventually leading to aphasia and inability to recognize even family members.

About 25 percent of cases can be due to genetic transmission. Amyloid precursor protein gene on chromosome 21 is responsible for early onset dementia. Chromosome 12 and E4 allele of apolipoprotein E (APOE-4) are responsible for late onset dementia. Tau protein and beta amyloid deposits are found to accumulate in the brain of Alzheimer's victims. One of the risk factors for Alzheimer's disease could be a variant of a certain gene called apolipoprotein E or known as APOE. Everyone has two copies of this gene, one inherited from each parent. It can have three variants. The e-4 variant is associated with heightened risk for Alzheimer's disease. It is estimated that 20 percent of the population has one such variant putting them at higher risk.

There are three abnormalities noted in the brain of patients with Alzheimer's disease. First is the accumulation of microscopic clumps of a protein called beta-amyloid, also called plaques in the brain. Second is a protein called tau that twists into microscopic fibers called tangles, which affects brain cell transports. Third is a protein called fyn, which when combined with beta amyloid causes destruction of synapses. Based on these facts, research is performed to develop drugs. Monoclonal antibodies have the promise of reducing amyloid plaques. Tau aggression inhibitors and tau vaccines are being studied in clinical trials. Another drug called sargramostim (Leukine) is in research and considered to stimulate the immune system and reduce the inflammatory process caused by the above proteins.

An extensive study was presented at the Alzheimer's Association International Conference in Los Angeles in July 2019, which showed that certain lifestyle changes could reduce risk of Alzheimer's disease by 60 percent. The report compiled by Rush University Medical Center in Chicago tracked 2,765 older persons over a decade. Five metrics were studied and followed: diet, exercise, smoking, alcohol intake, and cognitive stimulating activities.

Diet that is mostly vegetarian with nuts, berries, beans, whole grains, seafood, poultry, and olive oil, and avoiding red meat, butter, cheese, pastries, sweets, and fried food is beneficial. A small amount of alcohol in the form of red wine is thought to be acceptable. The MIND diet (Mediterranean-DASH Intervention for Neurodegenerative Delay) includes the above with extra leafy vegetables and berries and is found to reduce onset of Alzheimer's disease and dementia.

Exercise for at least 150 minutes per week, nonsmoking, and alcohol of only one glass of wine per day were beneficial. Exercise increases blood flow to the brain, raises levels of HDL cholesterol, and helps to form new synapses in the brain, protecting against brain cell death. Individuals also develop better memory and improve cognition. Studies show that regular aerobic exercise decreases tau protein in the spinal fluid, thus reducing the onset of dementia.

Mentally stimulating activities include reading, writing, or games such as chess, checkers, or crossword puzzles. These five lifestyle changes can reduce the risk of dementia and Alzheimer's disease. These lifestyle changes are to be started in midlife rather than waiting for old age since it takes many years for neurological changes to be detected.

Adequate sleep is considered a factor as well. No one really knows why we sleep, but it is common knowledge that we feel refreshed after a good night of sleep, and we perform our best work early in the morning. During sleep, the brain washes off toxic substances, including tau proteins and beta amyloids.

Approximately fifty million people worldwide have dementia. That number is expected to triple by 2050. The abovementioned lifestyle changes also helped genetically predisposed individuals to delay the development of Alzheimer's disease according to a study conducted by University of Exeter Medical School at the same time. Medications have been developed and tried to help these individuals but with minor improvement. Maintaining blood pressure control has been shown to decrease incidence of dementia and stroke. Smoking worsens their outcome in individuals predisposed.

The workup of these patients includes blood tests for routine medical problems, vitamin deficiencies, hormonal abnormalities, and renal problems. One must rule out infections, latent syphilis,

HIV/AIDS, and alcoholism. Imaging studies of MRI or CT scan is done to rule out intracranial lesions and vascular or hemorrhagic incidents. The hippocampus of the brain is found to shrink in those with Alzheimer's disease as seen in MRI studies. PET amyloid and tau imaging studies show enlargement of the ventricles with consequential reduction of brain volume.

Other tests are done to evaluate cognitive and mental status. A full neurological and physical examination is included to identify comorbidities and contributing factors and to assess the physical and mental status of the patient. Mini-Mental State Examination (MMSE) is a thirty-point test that evaluates recall, delayed recall, concentration, and language and visual spatial domains. Montreal cognitive assessment and mini-cog testing are similar cognitive tests. Kohlman evaluation of living skills is done to assess independent living ability of the individual. Genetic testing is done in research settings to assess the risk for Alzheimer's disease.

Medications available for treatment are: donepezil (Aricept), galantamine (Razadyne), rivastigmine (Exelon), memantine (Namenda), sertraline, risperidone, Zyprexa, Seroquel, ziprasidone, trazodone, and buspirone. However, so far, most medications have been ineffective in stopping or curing Alzheimer's disease. Vitamin E and ginkgo biloba are claimed to be useful, but there is not strong data to support its use.

The family and caregivers' roles cannot be underestimated. Concern for the safety of individuals with dementia is essential, such as avoiding driving, wandering, or traveling. Constant supervision at home is highly recommended for the individual's safety. Caregivers are to avoid confrontations and agitations as much as possible by understanding that these individuals lack impulse control and are uninhibited. The suggestions are to maintain familiarity and routines as much as possible, to reduce the number of choices and options given to them, to avoid asking them questions but just tell them what to do next, and to not try logic or reason since they cannot understand. Keep the big picture of their safety and comfort in mind and let them be themselves.

Table 15

Medications for dementia

Cholinesterase inhibitors:
Donepezil (Aricept) 5 mg per day
Galantamine ((Razadyne) 4 mg q twelve hours
Rivastigmine (Exelon) 3–6 mg q twelve hours

NMDA antagonist:
Memantine (Namenda) 5 mg per day
Memantine (Namenda XR) 7 mg per day
Namzaric (combination of donepezil and memantine)
Neurontin (Horizant, Gabapentin) 300 mg PO (not typically used for dementia)

Table 16

Medications for agitation

Agitation due to psychosis: (*not recommended for patients over sixty-five years old*)
Aripiprazole (Abilify) 2.5–12.5 mg/day
Olanzapine (Zyprexa, Zydis) 2.5–10 mg/day
Quetiapine (Seroquel) 12.5–100 mg per day
Risperidone (Risperdal) 0.25–3 mg per day

Agitation due to depression:
Citalopram (Celexa) 10–20 mg/day

Agitation because of irritability:
Buspirone (BuSpar) 15–60 mg per day
Trazodone (Desyrel) 50–100 mg per day

Agitation and aggression:
Carbamazepine (Tegretol) 300–600 mg per day
Divalproex sodium (Depakote, Epival) 500–1,500 mg/day
Olanzapine (Zyprexa) 2.5–5 mg IM
Lorazepam (Ativan) 1 ml, 2 mg, 4 mg IM, IV, 0.5–2 mg PO

Diazepam (Diastat, Valium, Dizac) Benzodiazepine 2–10 mg PO or IM/IV

Sexual aggression:
Estrogen (Premarin) 0.625–1.25 mg/day
Medroxyprogesterone (Depo-Provera) 100 mg IM/week
Leuprolide acetate (Lupron Depot) 7.5 mg IM per month

Table 17

Medications for treatment of psychosis

Second-generation antipsychotics:
(*not recommended for patients over sixty-five years old*)
(*Serotonin dopamine receptor antagonists*)
Aripiprazole (Abilify) 2–5 mg/day
Asenapine (Saphris) 5–10 mg q twelve hours
Clozapine (Clozaril) 25–150 mg/day
Iloperidone (Fanapta) 1–2 mg q twelve hours
Lurasidone (Latuda) 40 mg/day
Olanzapine (Zyprexa) 2.5–10 mg/day
Paliperidone (Invega) 3–12 mg/day
Quetiapine (Seroquel) 25–800 mg/day
Risperidone (Risperdal) 0.25–1.0 mg/day
Ziprasidone (Geodon) 20–80 mg/day

First-generation antipsychotics:
(*not recommended for patients over sixty-five years old*)
(*D2 antagonists*)
Thioridazine (Mellaril) 25–200 mg/day
Perphenazine (Trilafon) 2–32 mg/day
Haloperidol (Haldol) 0.5–2 mg/day
Fluphenazine 1–2.5 mg/day
Adasuve (Loxitane) 5–50 mg/day

For ADHD, psychostimulant, narcolepsy:
Dexedrine (dextroamphetamine sulfate, Liquadd, Procentra, Zenzedi) 5 mg PO

Parkinson's disease

Parkinson's disease is a slowly progressive neurodegenerative disease, where there is loss of pigmented neurons in substantia nigra and brain stem and presence of Lewy bodies (concentric hyaline cytoplasmic inclusions). Patients have bradykinesia, rigidity, dystonia, tremors, pill rolling movements, and gait impairment. Associated symptoms include hypophonia, micrographia, depression, drooling, constipation, and seborrheic dermatitis. Hypotension, dementia, and sleep disorders can occur.

Bradykinesia is slowness or lack of movement with loss of dexterity and difficulty in making movements such as eating or dressing.

In moderate Parkinson's disease, there is gait dysfunction. Initially, there is shortened stride length and decreased arm swing with a stooping posture. Later, gait becomes shuffling steps, and the body turns en bloc, requiring several steps to make a turn. Treatment includes Levodopa 300–500 mg/day with carbidopa 75 mg/day (Duodopa). Other medications of use are pramipexole, bromocriptine (Parlodel), pergolide (Permax), selegiline (Deprenyl), COMT (Catechol O methyltransferase inhibitors), propranolol, anticholinergics amantadine, and Clozapine (Clozaril).

Stereotactic pallidotomy is done to control the tremors and symptoms. Deep brain stimulation (DBS) is a four-contact lead implanted on both sides of the brain by stereotactic technique, and the leads are connected to a pulse generator implanted in a subcutaneous plane in the chest wall.

Team management with care support, protein-restricted diet, and symptom relief is needed. Exercises and rehabilitation with emotional and religious support are helpful. A well-balanced, healthy diet with protein restriction with adequate hydration can reduce chances for constipation and hypotension. Amino acids compete with levodopa for absorption, thus blocking the therapeutic effect of medication.

Sleep disorders

Considering the many potential adverse health effects of insufficient sleep, it is not surprising that poor sleep is associated with lower life expectancy.

While an estimated 50 to 70 million Americans suffer from some type of sleep disorder, most people do not mention sleeping problems to their doctors, and most doctors do not routinely ask about them. This widespread lack of awareness of the impact of sleep problems can have serious and costly public health consequences.

Health professionals now recommend paying attention to sleep hygiene as well as all other aspects of sleep to improve health and well-being.

These disorders and the resulting sleep deprivation interfere with work, driving, and social activities. They also account for an estimated $16 billion in medical costs each year while the indirect costs due to lost productivity and other factors are probably much greater.

Insomnia

Everyone occasionally suffers from short-term insomnia. Problems can result from stress, jet lag, diet, and other factors. Insomnia always affects job performance and well-being, especially on the day after a restless night.

About sixty million Americans per year have insomnia at any given time. Simple insomnia can lead to even more serious sleep deficits.

Insomnia increases with age, starting in our late teenage years, and worsens over time. Insomnia affects about 40 percent of women and 30 percent of men. It is often the major disabling symptom of an underlying medical disorder. Such disorders can be hiatal hernia with acid reflux, obesity, alcoholism, stress, intake of certain medications, infections, chronic pain, urinary retention, and sleep apnea syndrome.

For short-term insomnia, doctors may prescribe sleeping pills. Most sleeping pills stop working after just a few weeks of nightly use; however, long-term use can create dependency and can interfere with good sleep.

Mild insomnia is preventable or cured by practicing good sleep habits.

Sleep apnea

Sleep apnea is a disorder that results in interrupted breathing during sleep. It usually occurs in conjunction with the fat buildup or the loss of muscle tone that comes with aging. These changes allow the windpipe to collapse during breathing when muscles relax during sleep.

We usually associate obstructive sleep apnea with loud snoring, although not everyone who snores has the disorder. Sleep apnea can also occur if the neurons that control breathing malfunction during sleep.

During an episode of obstructive apnea, the person's effort to inhale air creates suction, which collapses the windpipe. This can block the airflow for ten seconds up to a minute while the sleeping person struggles to breathe. When the person's blood oxygen level falls, the brain responds by waking the person just enough to tighten the upper airway muscles and open the windpipe. The person may snort or gasp then resume snoring. This cycle repeats itself hundreds of times a night.

The frequent awakening that patients with sleep apnea experience can leave them continually sleepy and may lead to personality changes such as irritability or depression. Sleep apnea also deprives the person of oxygen. Such deprivation can lead to morning headaches, a loss of interest in sex, or a decline in mental functioning. Sleep apnea is linked to high blood pressure, irregular heartbeats, and an increased risk of heart attacks and stroke.

Patients with severe, untreated sleep apnea are two to three times more likely to have automobile accidents than the general population. In high-risk individuals, sleep apnea may even lead to sudden death from respiratory arrest during sleep.

An estimated eighteen million Americans have sleep apnea. However, few have had the problem diagnosed. Patients who show the typical features of sleep apnea—such as loud snoring, obesity, and excessive daytime sleepiness—warrant referred to a specialized sleep center where a test called polysomnography, also known as a sleep study, can be performed.

It is possible for individuals to overcome mild sleep apnea by losing weight or by not sleeping on his or her back. Other sufferers may need special devices or surgery to correct the obstruction.

People with sleep apnea should never take sedatives or sleeping pills, which can prevent them from awakening enough to breathe. In other words, they could suffer severe injury to their nervous system. They could even die.

Restless legs syndrome

Restless legs syndrome (RLS) is a familial disorder that causes unpleasant crawling, prickling, or tingling sensations in the legs and feet and an urge to move them for relief. It is appearing as one of the most common sleep disorders, especially among older people, often starting after age fifty. Current treatment options include the following:
- Medicines used to treat Parkinson's disease.
- Medications that increase dopamine in the brain (rotigotine [Neupro] and pramipexole [Mirapex]). These medications affect the levels of the chemical messenger dopamine in the

brain. Short-term side effects of these medications are usually mild and include nausea, lightheadedness, and fatigue. However, they can also cause impulse control disorders such as compulsive gambling and daytime sleepiness.

- Drugs affecting calcium channels. Certain medications such as gabapentin (Neurontin, Gralise), gabapentin enacarbil (Horizant), and pregabalin (Lyrica) work for some people with RLS.
- Muscle relaxants and sleep medications. These drugs help you sleep better at night, but they do not eliminate the leg sensations and may cause daytime drowsiness. These medications are only used if no other treatment provides relief.

Epilepsy

Epilepsy is excessive and abnormal neuronal activity leading to convulsive involuntary muscle contractions. In certain situations, it can be non convulsive with decreased level of consciousness or brief undetectable focal seizures. Most cases of epilepsy disorders are discovered in young individuals and may have a genetic etiology. In the older individuals, one may notice acquired causes such as trauma, stroke, tumors, infections, toxemia or medications. Treatment is mostly by use of anticonvulsant drugs and correction of underlying causes.

Seizures in older adults often are often overlooked and are subtler than those experienced by younger people; therefore, patients, caregivers, and even physicians may not detect them. Diagnosing and treating seizures in older adults is imperative because it could stave off cognitive decline.

One in four newly diagnosed patients with epilepsy in the US is sixty-five or older and many who have seizures in that age range are not diagnosed. Stroke is the most common cause of seizures in older adults. A patient with a new-onset seizure who has not experienced a stroke has an elevated risk of doing so within four weeks of their first seizure.

Alzheimer's disease and Lewy body dementia also have a complicated association with seizures. Both are risk factors for seizures, but sometimes, treating the seizures limits the dementia symptoms.

Older adults who have seizures often experience focal seizures—brief staring spells without muscle movements or convulsions. One can confuse a brief spell of inattention in an older person with a memory lapse or even a transient ischemic attack. An older adult who has periods of inattention should be evaluated for the potential of seizures. An EEG might be helpful in sorting out the cause but is not always a reliable tool in older patients.

Chapter 13

Gastrointestinal Disorders

Common gastrointestinal problems affecting older adults are indigestion, heartburn, dysphagia, peptic ulcer disease, constipation and fecal impaction, diarrhea, cancer of colon and rectum, diverticulitis, and fecal incontinence.

Indigestion/dyspepsia

Indigestion/dyspepsia is a symptom conglomerate with many potential causes and the patient describes it as stomach upset. It could be food allergy, food poisoning, peptic ulcer disease and acute gastritis, excess intake of alcohol or analgesics, or hiatal hernia.

Efforts are made to find the initiating cause-and-stop continuation of the same. Often medications such as Pepto-Bismol or Alka-Seltzer are used. Cessation of NSAIDS and alcohol is recommended.

Heartburn / hiatal hernia

Reflux esophagitis with acid regurgitation and reflux of undigested food into the mouth are associated with sliding hiatal hernia, where lower esophageal sphincter is above the diaphragm and the esophageal hiatal opening is patulous. Barrett's esophagus has columnar epithelium in the lower esophagus, which can mutate to malignancy.

Patients present with symptoms of heartburn or substernal pain with radiation to mouth and throat after meals, especially following spicy meals, tomato paste, or alcohol. There is regurgitation of food often with sour taste. Sometimes the patients have atypical symptoms, such as sudden waking up from sleep, chronic cough, or laryngitis. Patients experience relief from milk and alkaline medications such as Alka-Seltzer.

Investigations should include upper endoscopy and biopsy of the lower esophageal mucosa, twenty-four-hour pH monitoring and esophageal manometry. These will rule out Barrett's esophagus, confirm presence of acid reflux, and confirm patulous lower esophageal sphincter. An upper GI series with esophageal study will also visualize the anatomy.

Complications and sequelae may include lower esophagitis, bleeding, anemia, stricture formation and dysphagia, and malignant transformation. Acid reflux could be one of the symptoms of sleep disorders.

Treatment with medical measure with surgery as a later option. Having a bland diet, eating slowly in small quantities, sitting in erect or semierect posture after eating, walking after eating, and sleeping with pillows are conservative measures. Medications such as Pepcid, Protonix, Prilosec, Prevacid, or AcipHex are useful.

Surgery aims to bring the lower esophageal sphincter below the diaphragm and create a wrap around the lower esophagus as in Nissen fundoplication. The intra-abdominal pressure as well as the intraluminal pressure tightens the lower esophagus and controls the reflux. If Barrett's esophagus is noted, one should look for evidence of metaplasia or neoplasia in the lower esophagus. If so, the patient will require aggressive intervention to prevent carcinoma.

Peptic ulcer disease (PUD)

Mucosal ulcerations of the stomach and duodenum are usually due to bacterial infestation by Helicobacter pylori. Previously, PUD was attributed to excess hydrochloric acid in the stomach. Other causes are side effects of NSAIDs or aspirin and alcohol abuse, Zollinger-Ellison syndrome, a retained antrum, previous gastric surgery, G-cell hyperplasia, hyperparathyroidism, sepsis, instrumentations and irritation by prolonged nasogastric intubation, head injury, major trauma, and multiple organ failure. Gastric ulcers can be due to cancers or stromal tumors.

Diagnosis of the ulcer is by upper endoscopy. Various gastric acid studies have been abandoned. Endoscopic biopsy and urea breath tests will be adequate to confirm H. pylori infection. Complications of untreated peptic ulcer disease include bleeding, perforation, continued abdominal pain, and dyspepsia, leading to nutritional deficiencies.

Medical treatment for H. pylori infection is antibiotics: clarithromycin 500 mg every twelve hours and amoxicillin 1,000 mg every twelve hours for two weeks. Metronidazole 500 mg every twelve hours is another possibility if allergic to penicillin. Along with this, antacids or proton pump inhibitors are used. For gastric ulcers, sucralfate along with H2 antagonists or PPIs are used. Prevention also involves reducing stress, alcohol, aspirin, and NSAIDs. In cases of gastric ulcers, malignancy must be ruled out with endoscopic biopsy.

Surgery is needed if medical treatment fails or if complications such as perforation, severe bleeding, or pyloric stenosis occur. This involves correcting the immediate problem, such as obstruction, bleeding, or perforation. An acid-reducing procedure is contemplated, but infrequently. Such procedures could be truncal vagotomy, pyloroplasty, partial gastrectomy, or subtotal gastrectomy. If malignancy is discovered, adequate margin clearing gastrectomy is done. Suitable reconstructions are done such as Billroth 1 or Billroth 2 or Roux en Y reconstructions.

Table 18

Medications of use in acid reflux, peptic ulcer, stress ulcer

Antacids:
Mylanta
Maalox
Gaviscon
Tums
Rolaids
Pepto-Bismol
Alka-Seltzer

Histamine-2 receptor blockers:
Cimetidine (Tagamet) 300–600 mg PO four times a day
Famotidine (Pepcid) 10–40 mg PO
Nizatidine (Axid) 300 mg PO

Proton pump inhibitors:
Esomeprazole (Nexium) 20–40 mg PO
Lansoprazole (Prevacid) 15 mg PO/day
Omeprazole (Prilosec) 20 mg PO/day
Pantoprazole (Protonix) 40 mg PO or IV per day
Rabeprazole (AcipHex) 20 mg/day

Antibiotics against H. pylori:
Clarithromycin (Biaxin) 500 mg PO
Amoxicillin 250–500 mg PO
Metronidazole 500 mg PO

Others:
Sucralfate (Carafate) 1 mg PO as a tablet or solution

Diarrhea

Diarrhea can be due to acute infectious conditions such as food poisoning, or infections such as salmonella, shigella, or cholera. Long-standing and recurrent diarrhea is often due to inflammatory bowel disorders such as ulcerative colitis, Crohn's disease, or short gut syndrome. Following hospitalization and antibiotic therapy, one can develop clostridium difficile infection and pseudomembranous colitis. Steatorrhea can be due to pancreatic insufficiency. Resection of terminal ileum leads to lack of bile salt reabsorption leading to diarrhea. Bariatric surgical procedures or resections of bowel or colon can lead to diarrhea. Diarrhea is also reported after vagotomy and cholecystectomy. Medications and certain foods can have a laxative effect. Irritable bowel syndrome presents with episodes of abdominal discomfort, constipation, and diarrhea. Ischemic bowel can lead to bloody stools and diarrhea. Lactose intolerance, food allergies, and malabsorption syndromes are also causes of diarrhea.

Acute infectious diarrhea may need IV fluids to avoid dehydration and antibiotic coverage. Binding agents are Kaopectate, Pepto-Bismol, Imodium, and Lomotil (Lonox) (atropine sulfate / diphenoxylate) 5 mg four times a day. For the loss of the ileal reabsorption of bile salts, one may try cholestyramine. Clostridium difficile colitis is treated with full isolation precautions. All antibiotics are stopped, and the patient is given vancomycin and metronidazole orally. Newer agents to treat clostridium difficile include Fidaxomicin. These patients need close monitoring to make sure they do not transition into toxic megacolon. If a patient develops a toxic megacolon with impending perforation or real perforation, the patient will need emergency surgery. This may involve subtotal colectomy with ileostomy. An alternative possibility is an ileostomy and lavage of the colon with glycolic solution and vancomycin.

Constipation

Fecal is one of the common problems faced by the very older adult and bedridden individuals. There is a loss of motility of the colon due to neuromuscular dysfunction. Oral intake of fiber in food may not be adequate, thus reducing the bulk. Body biorhythms can change with bedridden status. Continued fecal impaction can result in secondary abdominal distension, partial or complete bowel obstruction, an acquired megacolon, and even perforation of caecum. Other factors could be central nervous system disorders, such as CVA, Parkinson's disease, and dementia. Use of certain medications such as iron, anticholinergics, calcium channel blockers, narcotics, and diuretics can cause constipation. Finally, one should not ignore the possibility of malignancy and obstructive lesions in the older adult.

The physician should evaluate all patients to make sure one is not missing a cancer of the colon or rectum. Complete physical examination, including rectal examination, is needed. Change in bowel habits and hemoccult positive stool should raise the suspicion of cancer. X-ray of the abdomen, CT scan, and colonoscopy are tests of value.

Prevention of constipation in older adults includes adequate intake of fluids and fiber diet, ambulation, maintaining normal bowel habits, and use of Metamucil, Benefiber, or Citrucel. Further care may involve use of mild laxative or stool softeners such as Surfak or Colace, milk of magnesia, or Dulcolax.

Once a fecal impaction is diagnosed, disimpaction by manual measures followed by oral laxatives or enemas with oil or saline is administered. If further damage is noted with a megacolon or impending perforation, surgery may be necessary. This may involve colostomy or colectomy. If cancer is discovered by investigations, then appropriate surgery to resect the malignancy is recommended.

Table 19

Medications of use in constipation

Bulking agents:
Psyllium
Calcium polycarbophil
Methyl cellulose (Metamucil, Citrucel)

Stool softeners:
Docusate calcium / sodium (Surfak, Colace)
Mineral oil

Osmotic laxatives:
Lactulose
Sorbitol
Polyethylene glycol (Colyte, Golytely)
Magnesium hydroxide/sulfate

Miralax

Stimulants:
Senna
Bisacodyl
Dulcolax

Serotonin agonists:
Tegaserod maleate
Prucalopride

Chloride channel activator:
Lubiprostone

Guanylate cyclase-C receptor antagonists:
Linaclotide

Probiotics:
Lactobacillus
Bifidobacterium

Malnutrition

Older adults are likely to suffer from malnutrition for multiple reasons. They lack interest in eating and have diminished appetites. Dementia, poverty, poor dentures, lack of caregivers, inadequate attention, dyspepsia, chronic illnesses, and malabsorption are other factors. The patient may lose weight, get dehydrated, and may develop vitamin and trace metal deficiencies. Treatment is with adequate hydration and support of full nutrition and supplemental vitamins and minerals. At times pureed food is necessary or tube feeding may have to be initiated.

Diverticulitis of colon

Etiology of the diverticulum of the colon is still unclear. It could be genetic predisposition, constipation, or low-residue diet that leads to protrusion of the mucosa through the wall of the colon. It is less common in the Eastern hemisphere, where the people eat a high-fiber diet and have easier bowel habits in a squatting position. Once the diverticulum has formed, it is prone to microperforation of the mucosa, resulting in inflammation, abscess formation, or free perforation. The diverticula can also cause rectal bleeding. Most episodes of diverticular bleedings cease spontaneously. If bleeding persists, surgery to resect the involved segment of the colon is to be considered.

Symptoms vary depending on the extent of disease. Asymptomatic diverticula do not require any treatment. High-fiber diet and avoiding nuts are recommended. Once mild inflammation occurs, there is pain and tenderness in the left lower quadrant of abdomen, along with fever and leukocytosis. IV antibiotics of broad-spectrum nature are administered. There is good recovery in most cases. In more severe forms with marked inflammation, one could administer IV antibiotics to control the sepsis and then plan for a one-stage resection and anastomosis of the involved segment. When a well-walled-off abscess is found, percutaneous drainage is done under CT guidance, and once the inflammation has cooled off, a one-stage resection and anastomosis is done. If the infection is very severe with acute peritonitis, the patient will need emergency laparotomy with resection of the involved segment and end colostomy and Hartman closure of distal stump. After a six-month interval, a second stage repair can be performed to reestablish bowel continuity. Most diverticular bleedings stop spontaneously. If the bleeding persists or if it is severe, then they will need surgery to resect the bleeding segment of the bowel.

Inflammatory bowel disease

Inflammatory bowel disease (IBD), including Crohn's disease (CD) and ulcerative colitis (UC), can develop at any age, including in older adults. It is expected that there will be increasing numbers of older adults with IBD, considering the demographic shift to aging populations. The care of aging patients with IBD poses unique challenges with respect to diagnosis and treatment options. Clinicians must be prepared to diagnose and initiate care for older patients despite underlying conditions. Common comorbidities include malignancies and increased disposition to infections, which can expose this more vulnerable age group to complications from immunosuppression.

IBD (CD, UC) presents in older patients with diarrhea, rectal bleeding, urgency, abdominal pain, or weight loss. Up to 15 percent of new diagnoses of IBD occur in individuals older than sixty years. Fecal calprotectin or lactoferrin may help prioritize patients with a low probability of IBD for endoscopic evaluation. In older patients with segmental left-sided colitis in the setting of diverticulosis, consideration includes the diagnosis of segmental colitis associated with diverticulosis in addition to the possibility of CD or UC.

A typical evaluation would include a comprehensive assessment of the older patient followed by the establishment of short- and long-term treatment goals and priorities.

Risk-stratification of patients is based on the likelihood of severe clinical course, including an assessment of perianal or penetrating phenotype, long-segment small bowel involvement (CD), extensive colitis (UC), anemia, hypoalbuminemia, elevated inflammatory markers, and weight loss.

Systemic corticosteroids are not indicated for maintenance therapy. When used for induction therapy, clinicians should prefer nonsystemic corticosteroids (like budesonide) or even early biological therapy initiation. The criteria for immunosuppression should be based on chronologic age as well as considering the patient's functional status, comorbidities (including prior neoplasia and potential for infectious complications), and frailty.

When possible, immunotherapy treatments such as vedolizumab or ustekinumab may be preferred in older adults, since they carry lower risk for infection or malignancy. Consideration of thiopurine monotherapy for the maintenance of remission in older patients should balance the convenience of its oral route of administration and lower cost with lower efficacy, slow onset of action, and an increase in risk of nonmelanoma skin cancers and lymphoma in this population.

As surgery is sometimes a choice, the type and timing in older patients with IBD should incorporate disease severity as well as the impact on functional status and independence.

The increased risk of fracture, venous thromboembolism, infections (including pneumonia, opportunistic infections, and herpes zoster), and the risk of skin and nonskin cancers (including lymphoma) should be incorporated in the therapeutic decision process.

Care for the older patient with IBD should be multidisciplinary, actively engaging gastrointestinal specialists, primary care providers (including geriatricians), other medical subspecialists, mental health professionals, general or colorectal surgeons, nutritionists, and pharmacists. Engaging with family and caregivers may also be appropriate in formulating a plan.

Chapter 14
Hepatobiliary and Pancreatic Disorders

Liver diseases

Cirrhosis of the liver is the most common liver disease affecting older adults. Alcohol abuse, congestive heart failure, and metabolic and nutritional problems take a toll on the liver, which develops scar tissue and cicatrix, causing portal hypertension, ascites, and hepatic insufficiency. Patients present with jaundice, ascites, hematemesis, malnutrition, failure to thrive, and coagulopathy. Liver function tests and liver biopsy are confirmatory. Treatment is mostly supportive care in the early stage, correcting metabolic and nutritional deficiencies. Once advanced portal hypertension is established, a portosystemic shunt using the noninvasive method called TIPS procedure (transjugular intrahepatic portosystemic shunt) is considered.

Other liver diseases are hepatitis A, B, and C, parasitic infections such as amoebiasis, hydatid disease, malaria, and schistosomiasis. Liver abscess can be bacterial or parasitic in origin. Metastatic malignancy and primary malignancy of the liver can occur. Primary cancers of the liver are hepatoma or hepatocellular carcinoma and cholangiocarcinoma. Metastatic malignancy is usually from the GI tract, mostly colorectal in origin or from breast, lung, or hematological.

Nonalcoholic fatty liver (NAFLD) has been shown to be a major contributor to chronic liver disease and cirrhosis. It is treated with diet management, particularly reduction in sugar and carbohydrate intake.

Biliary system disorders

Gallstones and associated problems are common. Initially, they present as dyspepsia, right upper quadrant abdominal pain, and discomfort. When acute cholecystitis occurs, the patient develops fever, abdominal pain, and tenderness with leukocytosis. These patients will need laparoscopic cholecystectomy. If there is evidence of acute cholecystitis, they are started on IV antibiotics. In all these cases, besides a routine CBC and liver chemistries; serum amylase and lipase levels are run to detect common bile duct stones and biliary pancreatitis. Ultrasound of the abdomen is the best test to diagnose gallstones. CT scan or MRCP (magnetic resonance cholangiopancreatography) is requested if liver chemistries are elevated. Such abnormal chemistries may show pancreatic lesions or common bile duct stones. If common bile duct stones are noted, then the choices are (a) to do preoperative ERCP and removal of the stone after papillotomy followed by laparoscopic cholecystectomy and (b) to address both gallstones and common duct stones at one sitting intraoperatively either by open surgery or by laparoscopic method. If the common duct stones are diagnosed during cholecystectomy while doing an intraoperative cholangiogram, one may remove those stones at the same sitting or have them removed postoperatively using ERCP technique. Older bedridden patients or otherwise ill patients can develop acute cholecystitis without gallstones. It is referred to as acalculous cholecystitis. One may do a percutaneous cholecystostomy if the patient is acutely ill or debilitated to undergo cholecystectomy. If there is evidence of pancreatitis, cholecystectomy is delayed until the pancreatitis has cooled off.

Acute pancreatitis

Acute hemorrhagic pancreatitis is a chemical burn of the retroperitoneum resulting in marked abdominal pain, dehydration, shock, and metabolic changes. Patients may deteriorate into multiple organ failure with resultant death if not treated aggressively. The exact etiology is often unknown. Small stones in the ampulla of Vater or instrumentation such as ERCP (endoscopic retrograde cholangiopancreatography) can precipitate one. Alcohol intake and nutritional factors are considered. Bacterial infection is not a cause, at least in the initial period. The pancreas gets swollen and edematous with marked inflammatory type reaction of the retroperitoneum. CT scan of abdomen is diagnostic and can also evaluate the severity of the reaction. Serum amylase and lipase levels are elevated and are the best diagnostic tools in the emergency room.

There can be a reduction in hematocrit and serum calcium, and the patient may develop metabolic acidosis. Intravascular dehydration occurs due to third spacing and capillary leak, and the patient may develop acute renal failure.

Treatment includes resting the pancreas by keeping the patient NPO (nothing per oral) along with administering intravenous fluid and while watching metabolic parameters.

Metabolic abnormalities will correct over time with good systemic support, and the acute inflammation should subside. Sequelae include formation of pancreatic abscesses, pseudo cyst formation or chronic pancreatitis, and diabetes mellitus.

Pancreatic cancer

Cancer of the head of the pancreas causes compression of distal common bile duct as it traverses through the head of pancreas, resulting in obstructive jaundice. Gallbladder and the extra hepatic biliary tree dilate and lack of bile in stool causes it to become clay colored. Gallbladder gets distended and becomes palpable as Courvoisier's gallbladder. Liver chemistries show elevated direct bilirubin and mildly elevated liver enzymes and alkaline phosphatase. CT scan of abdomen is diagnostic with a mass noted in the head of pancreas and dilatation of extra hepatic biliary tree. A percutaneous fine needle aspiration cytology of the mass can be done to confirm tissue diagnosis. If the mass is resectable, surgery by pancreaticoduodenectomy (Whipple resection) offers the best chance for a cure. If it is not resectable, a palliative bypass such as cholecystojejunostomy can be done to reduce the jaundice level. An alternative is the placement of a biliary stent by ERCP technique.

Chapter 15

Psychological Problems in Older Adults

Depression, mood swings, anxiety, dementia, alcohol abuse, drug abuse, schizophrenia, and suicidal tendencies are psychological problems affecting aging adults.

Depression

Depression is described as having a depressed mood and loss of interest in all activities for at least two weeks, associated with such feelings as worthlessness, guilt, insomnia, diminished ability to concentrate or think, loss of appetite, and retardation.

Depression can be primarily related to aging and cerebral changes. Depression can be secondary to a medical condition such as diabetes mellitus, cerebrovascular problems, thyroid dysfunction, or medication effects. Other risk factors are divorce, bereavement, illnesses, disabilities, sleep disorders, financial problems, isolation, caregiving for a disabled partner, sexual dysfunction, and substance abuse, including alcohol intake. Uncorrected depression can lead to suicide, homicide, malnutrition, and aggravation of existing medical problems due to lack of care and attention.

The first line of treatment is social and family support, encouraging physical activities, and group activities. Visiting friends, church, or temple, shopping, dining out, joining health clubs, senior care centers, and intervention from mental health providers and social workers are useful tools.

Treatment includes antidepressants, antipsychotics, and other classes of medications. Psychiatric therapy and electroconvulsive therapy may be a necessary possibility. A list of medications follows.

Table 20

Medications of use in depression

SSRI (selective serotonin reuptake inhibitor):
Citalopram (Celexa) 10–20 mg/day

Escitalopram (Lexapro) 10 mg/day
Fluoxetine (Prozac) 5 mg–60 mg/day
Fluvoxamine (Luvax) 25 mg/hour
Paroxetine (Paxil) 10–40 mg/day (anticholinergic)
Sertraline (Zoloft) 25–200 mg/day
Trazodone 150 mg PO per day in divided doses

TCA (Tricyclic antidepressant):
Desipramine (Norpramin) 50–150 mg/day (anticholinergic)
Sinequan (Doxepin) 75 mg/day (anticholinergic)
Tofranil (Imipramine) 25 mg/day (anticholinergic)
Nortriptyline (Aventyl, Pamelor) 7-5150 mg/day (anticholinergic)
Amitriptyline (Elavil, Enova, Vanatrip, Equipto) 1--75 mg PO/
day (anticholinergic)

SNRI (serotonin norepinephrine reuptake inhibitor):
Duloxetine (Cymbalta) 40–60 mg/day
Venlafaxine (Effexor) 75–225 mg/day
Desvenlafaxine (Pristiq) 50 mg–400 mg/day

Others:
Bupropion (Wellbutrin) 75–150 mg q twelve hours
Levomilnacipran (Fetzima) 20–40 mg/day
Methylphenidate (Ritalin) 5–10 mg/day
Mirtazapine (Remeron) 15–45 mg/day
Vilazadone (Viibryd) 10–40 mg/day
Vortioxetine (Brintellix) 5–10 mg/day
Dextroamphetamine 5–60 mg PO/day
Modafinil (Provigil) 100–200 mg PO/day

Mood stabilizers:
Lamictal 25–100 mg/day
Depakote (Valproic acid) 750 mg PO/day
Carbamazepine (Tegretol) 200 mg PO/day
Lithium (Lithobid, Eskalith) 300 mg PO three times a day

Antipsychotics:
Risperidone 1–6 mg PO/day
Olanzapine 10 mg PO/day
Quetiapine 50 mg PO/day
Aripiprazole (Abilify) 10–15 mg PO/day

Anxiety

Anxiety can be a primary anxiety disorder or secondary to stress situations or due to drug withdrawals. It can be a comorbid condition with depression. Post-traumatic stress disorders can be a variant form of anxiety. Forms of phobias and panic conditions and obsessive-compulsive disorders make up further entities. Patients may show tachycardia, tremors, flushing, unsteadiness, syncope, insomnia, headaches, and varying symptoms of indigestion, irritable bowels, abdominal pain, and hyperventilation. Lab tests and radiology investigations will come back with no positive findings. Treatment involves identifying the root cause. Medications such as SSRIs, risperidone, buspirone, lorazepam, or temazepam are indicated when anxiety syndromes are severe.

Addictive disorders

The most predominant addictive disorders seen in healthcare are smoking, alcohol abuse, opioid and other chemical addictions.

Cigarette smoking is an addiction to nicotine combined with habit formation. It often starts as a method to overcome nervousness or boredom. Teenagers start the habit as "the cool thing to do." Recently e-cigarettes and vaping have become popular. The tobacco industry has a role in promoting the habit for profit. Other forms of tobacco use, such as cigars, chewing items or snuffing items, also produce similar adverse medical effects from nicotine. It is a mild stimulant but causes harm by accelerating the process of atherosclerotic disease, heart attacks, lung cancers, oral cancers, and other systemic cancers. Smoking cessation requires a concerted effort once the habit becomes established. Medical therapy along with group therapies, psychological support, nicotine patches, and nonaddictive chewable products are available.

Alcohol abuse is a chemical dependency from which recovery is difficult. Greater than 66 percent of alcoholics suffer from chronic alcoholism as a lifelong condition. While small amounts of alcohol such as red wine might have benefits in reducing atherosclerosis and heart attacks, this would not apply to individuals with dependency. Individuals with alcohol dependency drink several drinks throughout the day and suffer consequences. Serious side effects are progressive such as cirrhosis of liver, portal hypertension, ascites, esophageal varices, hematemesis, and liver failure resulting in death.

It also causes permanent neurological damage with encephalopathy, dementia, delusions, and hallucinations. Nutritional deficiencies, gastritis, and cancers of visceral organs also occur. Alcohol dependence also leads to sexual dysfunction, depression, insomnia, and suicidal tendencies. It increases confusion, memory loss, ataxia, falls, and accidents. Wernicke's encephalopathy, acute delirium tremens, and seizures can occur during hospitalizations for acute withdrawal. Treatment includes rehabilitation and support. Organizations such as AA (Alcoholics Anonymous) are helpful in all stages of recovery. Detoxification requires patience, group therapy, and medications. Thiamine, oxazepam, lorazepam, Haldol, Antabuse (disulfiram), naltrexone, and ondansetron are various drugs useful depending on the situation. Patient education and family support are extremely important for successful recovery.

Substance use disorder includes dependence on a variety of substances such as opiates (heroin, oxycodone, hydrocodone, morphine, meperidine, cocaine, angel dust, fentanyl, ganja, and marijuana in various forms, synthetic drugs, LSD, and methamphetamine. Most of those affected are young, and only about 5 percent are older adults. Older adults often use diazepam, alprazolam, chlordiazepoxide, and other pain pills such as oxycodone, hydrocodone, or methadone. Chronic substance use leads to reduction in hepatic and renal function and causes constipation, dyspepsia, and neurological symptoms of mood changes, agitation, instability of gait, falls, confusion, erectile dysfunction, and diminished libido and overdose, resulting in respiratory or cardiac arrest. Blood tests such as drug panels are helpful in identifying the offending substance. Treatment includes gradual withdrawal, substitution with lower potent medications, group therapy and support groups, standard needle precautions, prevention of HIV/AIDs, safe sex practices, and treatment of overdose. Narcan has become well established and widespread to counteract opioid overdose. Symptomatic treatment of emesis, respiratory distress, seizures, and careful use of sedatives can be used as well.

By being aware of the risks and talking openly with healthcare providers, we can help older adults maintain their health and well-being.

Schizophrenia

Schizophrenia can be a new onset condition in the older adult, or it can be a long-standing psychotic illness. Manifestations are delusions, hallucinations, and disorganized or catatonic behavior.

Personality disorders, paranoid and obsessive-compulsive behavior, catatonic, disorganized, and distorted language and communication patterns are clinical features. Symptoms of visual or auditory hallucinations can occur in severe cases. CT scan and MRI show ventricular enlargement, cortical prominence, decreased temporal and hippocampal size, and increased basal ganglia size. Treatment includes antipsychotics, risperidone, quetiapine, or olanzapine. Nursing care and personal care are important to help these unfortunate victims. Behavioral therapy in a stable environment after acute episodes are stabilized. Structured programs and family supervision are helpful.

Chapter 16

Infections in the Older Adults

Older adults are more prone to various infections, and they have less ability to fight the infections because of diminished immune capacity. Infections can affect any part of the body, as in lung infections causing pneumonia and bronchitis, urinary tract infections, skin and soft tissue infections, infections related to implanted devices, vascular problems related to arterial or venous insufficiencies, gastrointestinal infections, viral infections, and cerebral infections. Older adults require active surveillance to diagnose and treat them early on to avoid further morbidity and mortality.

Lung infections

The incidence of pneumonia and chronic bronchitis increases with age. Asthma and bronchiectasis worsen with age. Tuberculosis reactivation occurs due to decreased immune system. Influenza is a widespread problem, and flu vaccines are recommended every year since there may be different mutations each year. One consequence of aging is a diminished capacity to cough up the sputum due to muscle weakness, which can lead to mucous plugs, causing collapse of segments of the lung. Older adults tend to aspirate food, vomitus, and saliva due to mild cerebrovascular incidents, dementia, bedridden status, and swallowing problems. The aspirated materials cause both chemical and bacterial reactions. Patients develop fever, cough, sweating, shortness of breath, and tachycardia. X-ray chest is diagnostic in most cases. They may need bronchoscopic aspiration and lavage, IV antibiotics, postural therapy, and chest physiotherapy. Pneumonia can be fatal in older patients.

Urinary tract infections (UTI)

Females are more prone to UTIs because of a shorter urethra than male counterparts. Repeated instrumentations and catheterizations are causes. Diabetes mellitus is a predisposing condition as well as benign hypertrophy of prostate, chronic prostatitis, urinary stones, anatomic weakening of pelvic floor, ascending pyelonephritis, chronic cystitis, fecal incontinence, neurological disorders such as CVA, Alzheimer's disease, and dementia leading to retention of urine. Patients develop fever, chills, dysuria, hematuria, suprapubic pain, and back pain. E. coli is the predominant bacterial organism. Other bacteria include proteus mirabilis, Pseudomonas aeruginosa, klebsiella, Enterobacter, and Serratia. Urine culture and blood culture are diagnostic. Urinalysis will show WBCs and bacteria. Patients usually respond to oral antibiotics, but severe or resistant infections may require intravenous antibiotics. Investigations include ultrasound of bladder and kidneys. Relapsing UTIs is a frequent problem, and efforts can be undertaken to correct the predisposing condition.

Skin and soft tissue infections

Soft tissue infections can be related to diabetes mellitus, arterial insufficiency, venous insufficiency, lowered immunity, increased risk for trauma and fall, allergic reactions and drug interactions, and exposure to sun and environmental hazards. Staphylococcus or streptococcus bacteria can cause these infections, but others are due to MRSA (methicillin-resistant staphylococcus aureus) infection and can be more difficult to treat.

Diabetes mellitus causes neurological damage to the peripheral nerve endings, resulting in neuropathy, loss of pain sensation, and trophic changes to joints. In addition, there is microvascular occlusion and decreased immunity, leading to necrosis of tissues and rapid progression of the infection with minimal external signs even from minor injuries. Necrotizing fasciitis and soft tissue infections occur in the lower extremities with wet gangrene. They can also present as diabetic carbuncles or deep-seated abscesses. Early recognition, wide debridement and drainage, and broad-spectrum antibiotic therapy are part of the treatment protocol. All devitalized tissues must be sharply debrided and deep cultures taken. The patient may need repeated debridement procedures.

Atherosclerotic peripheral vascular disease is more common in aging patients. Minimal injuries such as nail paring can progress to gangrene of a toe, which further advances to full gangrene of the foot requiring below-knee or above-knee amputations. Revascularization with endovascular or open technique in a prompt fashion can save the tissues.

Chronic venous insufficiency and varicose veins can cause ulcers and nonhealing wounds in the lower extremities. The deep venous system valves are incompetent, resulting in lymphedema, secondary varicosities, and induration of subcutaneous tissue. The tissues become firm, skin becomes dry, and itching causes small skin ulcerations. These get infected with strep and staph organisms, resulting in loss of skin from spreading subcutaneous infection. Varicose veins can also cause venous ulcers from venous stasis. Surgical procedures such as stripping and ligation, endovascular ablation of the varicose veins, and subfascial ligations of the perforator veins are treatment options. Deep vein insufficiency is a challenging problem. It is important to avoid dryness of skin and to avoid scratching. Moisturizing skin creams and early aggressive treatment of skin infections can avoid larger deep wounds.

Infections related to devices

Various devices are implanted or inserted for monitoring or controlling illnesses. Most are placed out of necessity; others are optional. Their number increases with age, and any of them can get infected and lead to more procedures, leading to extended hospitalization and prolonged antibiotic therapy.

Examples of implanted devices are central line or peripherally introduced central line (PICC line), a common step in hospitals. It provides access to the intravenous route to administer medications, fluids, and nutritional products. For someone with poor peripheral veins, it is extremely helpful. However, they can easily get infected, causing fever and bacteremia, requiring the catheter to be removed, and an alternate intravenous access established along with prolonged antibiotic therapy. Similar devices are Infusaport or Mediport, dialysis catheters, pacemakers, AICDs, insulin pumps and morphine pumps.

Hemodialysis accesses using synthetic grafts can get infected after repeated punctures. Vascular grafts, meshes implanted for hernia repair, or orthopedic implants can get infected. Some cases require major corrective surgery after removing the original implants. Prolonged antibiotic therapy with consultation from an infectious disease consultant is needed. Any course of antibiotic, long or short, can lead to clostridium difficile infection, requiring new antibiotic therapy and further surgery.

Decubitus ulcers (pressure ulcers)

Older patients are often bedridden and unable to turn around or ambulate. As a result, pressure sores develop on the presacral region, trochanteric region, and back. These are areas of contact with the bed. Blood supply becomes compromised in these areas because of constant pressure. Soft tissue necrosis occurs under the dermis, leading to sizable areas of skin breakdown resulting in secondary infections.

The medical team emphasizes risk assessment and preventive measures against decubitus ulcer development. Such measures include use of a water mattress, frequent turning of the body or ambulation, application of moisturizing cream with gentle massage of the pressure areas, and nutritional support. Early detection of redness or erythema or blister formation is imperative.

Once full thickness necrosis has occurred, adequate surgical debridement to excise all devitalized tissue is performed. Cultures of the deep wound bed are obtained, and appropriate antibiotics are administered. Wound care is a topic by itself, which requires dressing changes and, when appropriate, wound-vac application. Local agents include hydrogel, hydrocolloid, alginates, biomembranes, and saline-soaked gauze pads.

Coronavirus pandemic

A novel virus, COVID-19, led to a pandemic, affecting most countries and killing large numbers of people all over the world within the period of 2020–2023. Worldwide, thirty-one million people were infected, and 1.2 million died within the first ten months of the pandemic. At the time of this writing, January 2022, the worldwide total was 307 million infections and six million deaths, and in the United States there have been sixty-one million infections and over one million deaths.

Older individuals were most vulnerable to death because of lowered immunity, pre-existing medical conditions, and pre-existing pulmonary problems. It started in Wuhan, China, and rapidly spread throughout the world. The virus is a mutant form from an earlier flu-like virus SARS-2, comprising RNA covered by a thin layer of fat. The spread is by airborne method and from touch or contact with contaminated surfaces. It alters the cell membrane leading to destruction, especially the lung parenchyma.

During the first five days after contamination, patients exhibit no symptoms. This is the incubation period. However, during this time, they can contaminate others. Symptoms can be fever, dyspnea, coughing, sneezing, abdominal pain, nausea, loss of smell or taste for food, and myalgia or back pain. Eighty percent of infected patients with symptoms recover spontaneously after 7-14 days without medical treatment. The remaining twenty percent get worse and end up going to the hospital. Most of these hospitalized patients get well with supportive care. The remaining hospitalized patients require intensive care unit admission with the need for ventilator support. A substantial percentage of the admissions to ICU with the need for mechanical ventilation die within days of admission. Vaccines have been developed and administered in many countries throughout the world. In hospitals interventions are constantly evolving, and monoclonal antibody and antiviral medications are now available options. The best form of prevention is by taking precautions against contamination. Such measures include wearing a mask in public places, indoor places, or when in proximity to others, washing hands with soap and water frequently, using hand sanitizers as needed, avoiding touching the face or nose frequently, keeping at least six feet of distance from another person, avoiding crowded places, avoiding traveling, and essentially practicing self-isolation and social distancing as best as possible.

HIV

According to the Centers for Disease Control and Prevention (CDC), in 2018, over half of the individuals in the United States diagnosed with HIV were fifty or older.

This is the case because lifelong treatment with HIV medicines (antiretroviral therapy or ART) is helping people with HIV live longer, healthier lives. In addition, because of the effectiveness of these HIV medicines, there is an increasing number of older people who are living with HIV. Fresh cases of HIV are diagnosed in thousands of people aged fifty and older every year. HIV risk factors are the same for people of all age groups, but older adults are less likely to get tested.

Treatment of HIV with antiretroviral therapy is recommended for everyone with HIV. The choice of an HIV treatment regimen for older patients is based on the individual's needs.

Since older adults often have more comorbidities such as heart disease or cancer, options for HIV treatment can become complicated.

Risk factors for HIV are the same for the general population and for older adults, and in both groups, there may be a lack of awareness of HIV risk factors. In the US, risk factors include having anal or vaginal sex with someone who has an HIV infection without using a condom or who is taking medicines to prevent or treat HIV. A second risk is sharing injection drug equipment (e.g., needles) with someone who has HIV.

An age-related factor that puts older adults at risk for HIV is the thinning and dryness of vaginal tissue, which can cause tearing of the vagina during sex and lead to HIV transmission. This is complicated in that older adults are less likely to use condoms because of a lessened concern about pregnancy.

Recommendations for HIV testing include everyone from thirteen to sixty-four years of age at least once as part of routine care, and those at higher risk of HIV must get tested more often.

Older adults are less likely to get tested because they are thought to be at lower risk of getting HIV. As a result, health-care providers may not always think to test older people for HIV. Older adults may be embarrassed or afraid to be tested for HIV. Signs of HIV may be mistaken for symptoms of aging or of age-related conditions. Consequently, testing to diagnose the condition may not include HIV testing.

Current recommendations for treatment with HIV medicines include all patients with the infection. There are treatment regimens that take age into account and can be individualized.

Heart disease and cancer, which are more common among older adults, complicate HIV treatments. Side effects from HIV medicines and other medicines may occur more often in older people with HIV. In addition, there is an increased risk of drug interactions in an older person taking HIV medicines and medicines for other conditions. Cognitive changes can affect an older adult's ability to adhere to an HIV treatment regimen.

C. diff

Clostridium difficile is a gram-positive, spore-forming bacillus that causes disease following ingestion. In normal situations, the gut microbiome environment prevents/suppresses *C. difficile* from gaining a foothold in the intestine through colonization resistance. Systemic antibiotics disrupt the gut microbiome, making a patient vulnerable to a *C. difficile* infection. An epidemic strain of *C. difficile* emerged in 2005–2010, causing more severe disease, and it developed resistance to multiple antibiotics that had previously been effective.

C. difficile infection disproportionately affects older adults. Nearly 1 percent of all hospitalizations involve a *C. difficile* infection. C. difficile infections/colitis place a significant financial burden on health-care systems.

Antibiotic exposure and advanced age are the two greatest risk factors for a *C. difficile* infection. Gastric acid suppression (due to age or use of proton pump inhibitors) strongly correlates with *C. difficile* infections, although the mechanism is unclear. Most other risk factors reflect diminished health status (albumin ≤ 3.5 g/dl, underlying disease severity, and mechanical ventilation).

Older adults' frequent interactions with health-care systems increase their exposure to *C. difficile* spores. At-risk older adults often receive antibiotics, placing them at risk for *C. difficile* infection. With aging comes diet changes and immune senescence, and these changes lead to a less robust gut microbiome. A *C. difficile* infection may manifest with a range of symptoms including asymptomatic colonization, watery diarrhea, and fulminant colitis requiring colectomy. Older adults experience more severe disease and are at greater risk of recurrent disease. Metronidazole and oral vancomycin have been the mainstays of treatment. Fidaxomicin, while more expensive, reduces the likelihood of a first disease recurrence and is rapidly becoming a first-line choice due to the organism's resistance to metronidazole and vancomycin. Fecal transplant is an excellent therapy that is garnering greater attention.

C. difficile spores are difficult to remove using routine cleansing agents and may remain viable on environmental surfaces for months. Reducing the burden of *C. difficile* in the environment is critical in disease prevention. Health-care workers may serve as vectors; hand hygiene using soap and water is the best means to remove spores from their hands. Preventing unnecessary antimicrobial use through stewardship also reduces *C. difficile* infections.

Morbidity and mortality due to *C. difficile* is mostly iatrogenic. Fecal transplant centers may offer highly effective treatments for a *C. difficile* infection, particularly for recurrent episodes. Research efforts may lead to an effective, evidence-based probiotic therapy to treat a *C. difficile* infection.

Table 21

List of antibiotics

First-generation cephalosporin, good for gram-positive infections, commonly used as first line treatment:
Cefazolin (Ancef) 1 gm IV every eight hours
Cefalotin (Keflin) 1 gm IV every eight hours
Cefalexin (Keflex) 500 mg PO every six hours
Cefadroxil (Duricef) 1 gm IV every eight hours

Second-generation cephalosporin
Cefotetan (Cefotan) 1–2 gm IV every twelve hours

Cefuroxime (Ceftin) 1–2 gm IV every twelve hours

Third-generation cephalosporin, covers both gram-positive and gram-negatives except for pseudomonas:
Ceftazidime (Fortaz, Tazicef) 2 gm IV every eight hours
Ceftriaxone (Rocephin) 1–2 gm IV every eight hours
Cefotaxime (Claforan) 1–2 gm IV every eight hours

Fourth-generation cephalosporin
Maxipime (cefepime) 2 gm IV every eight hours

Penicillin, commonly used against gram positive, spirochetes, Lyme disease:
Ampicillin 1 gm IV every six hours
Amoxicillin 1 gm IV every six hours
Dicloxacillin 500 mg PO every eight hours
Methicillin 500 mg PO every eight hours
Nafcillin 1–2 GM IV every six hours
Ticarcillin 3.00 gm IV every eight hours
Penicillin G 1–2 gm IV every six hours
Oxacillin 1–2 gm IV q six hours

Penicillin combinations, gives broad-spectrum coverage:
Piperacillin/tazobactam (Zosyn) 3.375 gm IV q eight hours
Ticarcillin/clavulanate (Timentin) 3.1 gm IV q six hours
Ampicillin/sulbactam (Unasyn) 1-3 gm IV q eight hours
Amoxicillin/clavulanate (Augmentin) 500 mg PO q eight hours

Against streptococcal infections, upper respiratory infections:
Erythromycin (Erythrocin) 250-500 mg PO q eight hours
Azithromycin (Zithromax, Azasite, Z Pak, Zmax) 250–500 mg PO
Clarithromycin (Biaxin) 250 mg q eight hours
Roxithromycin 150–300 mg q eight hours
Daptomycin (Cubicin) 5 mg/kg q eight hours

Useful against methicillin-resistant infections (MRSA):
Linezolid (Zyvox) 10 mg/kg q eight hours
Daptomycin 5 mg/kg q eight hours
Doxycycline 500 mg PO q eight hours
Vancomycin 1 GM IV q twelve hours
Clindamycin (Cleocin) 150–300 mg q six hours

Tigecycline (Tygacil) 50 mg IV q twelve hours
Delafloxacin (Baxdela) 200 mg IV q twelve hours

Useful against bacteroides:
Clindamycin (Cleocin) 150–300 mg q six hours
Metronidazol (Flagyl) 500 mg PO q eight hours

Carbapenem: Broad spectrum coverage against gram positives and negatives
Imipenem/cilastatin (Primaxin) 500–1,000 mg IV q six hours
Ertapenem (Invanz) 1 gm IV q eight hours
Doripenem (Doribax) 500 mg IV q eight hours
Meropenem (Merrem) 500 mg IV q eight hours

Aminoglycosides, effective against gram-negative bacteria, such as E. coli, klebsiella, Pseudomonas aeruginosa:
Gentamicin 80 mg IV q eight hours
Kanamycin 500 mg IV q eight hours
Neomycin 1 gm–4 mg PO q six hours
Tobramycin 80 mg IV q eight hours
Amikacin 250 mg IV q eight hours

Synthetic broad-spectrum antibiotics:
Quinolones for GI infections, urinary infections, and respiratory infections
Ciprofloxacin (Cipro) 250–500 mg PO q twelve hours
Levofloxacin (Levaquin) 250–500 mg IV or PO q twelve hours
Gatifloxacin (Tequin) 400 mg IV q twelve hours

Sulfa drugs:
Sulfadiazine 2–4 gm PO/day
Sulfisoxazole (Gantrisin) 4gm PO/day
Sulfamethizole (Thiosul) 25 gm IV/day
Trimethoprim/sulfamethoxazole (Bactrim) 400/80 q twelve hours
Azactam (Aztreonam) 500 mg IV q twelve hours

Antifungal agents:
Fluconazol (Diflucan) 100 mg–150 mg IV q eight hours
Amphotericin (Abelcet) 5 mg/kg IV every twenty-four hours

Table 22

List of medications for other infections

For tuberculosis:
Streptomycin 1 gm q twelve hours for ten days
Rifampin (Rifadin) 600 mg q twelve hours
Ethambutol 15–25 mg/kg/day
Isoniazid (INH) 10–15 mg/kg/day
Pyrazinamide (Aldinamide) 40–45 mg/kg/day
Cycloserine (seromycin) 250–500 mg PO q twelve hours
Rifapentine (Priftin) 600 mg PO q twelve hours
Capreomycin (Capastat) 15–30 mg/kg/day

For leprosy:
Dapsone 100 mg PO
Clofazimine 100 mg PO per day

For parasitic infections (antihelminths):
Albendazole (Albenza) 200 mg tab times two
Mebendazole (Emverm) 500 mg PO single dose
Furoxone (furazolidone)

For urinary tract infections:
Cipro (ciprofloxacin)
Bactrim (trimethoprim-sulfamethoxazole)
Nitrofurantoin (Macrodantin)

For clostridium difficile:
Vancomycin
Metronidazole (Flagyl)
Fidaxomicin
For skin infections as topical agents:
Mafenide (Sulfamylon)
Silver sulfadiazine (Silvadene)
Neosporin ointment
Bacitracin ointment
Silver nitrate

Antiseptic solutions (for cleansing skin or wounds):
Betadine (povidone)
Mercurochrome
Chlorhexidine solution
Chloroxylenol
Octenidine dihydrochloride
Hydrogen peroxide solution
Isopropyl alcohol wipes, swabs, solution
Iodine (tincture of iodine)
Dakin's solution (sodium hypochlorite)
Saline irrigation or saline soaks

Table 23

Antiviral agents

Drugs for HIV/AIDS:
Abacavir (Ziagen)
Atazanavir (Reyataz)
Cobicistat (Tybost)
Didanosine (Videx)
Darunavir (Prezista)
Dolutegravir (Tivicay)
Emtricitabine (Emtriva)
Enfuvirtide (Fuzeon)
Efavirenz (Sustiva)
Etravirine (Intelence)
Fosamprenavir (Lexiva)
Indinavir (Crixivan)
Maraviroc (Selzentry)
Nevirapine (Viramune)
Ritonavir (Norvir)
Raltegravir (Isentress)
Rilpivirine (Edurant)
Stavudine (Zerit)
Tenofovir (Viread)
Zidovudine (Retrovir)

Drugs for Coronavirus:

Remdesivir
Monoclonal antibodies
Decadron
Anticoagulants
Paxlovid (Ritonavir) Pfizer
Lagevrio (Molnupiravir) Merck
Vaccines
    Moderna
    Pfizer
    Johnson & Johnson
    AstraZeneca
    Sputnik V
    Novavaxx

Drugs for herpes zoster:
Acyclovir 10 mg/kg IV for seven to twenty-one days depending on condition
Topical for herpes simplex / herpes vaginalis:
Docosanol (Abreva) 10 percent cream topical five times a day

Drugs for hepatitis C:
Harvoni
Viekira
Zapatier
Technivie
Epclusa
Vosevi
Mavyret
Paritaprevir
Simeprevir (Olysio)
Grazoprevir
Ledipasvir
Ombitasvir
Elbasvir
Sofosbuvir (Sovaldi)
Dasabuvir
Ribavirin (Copegus, Moderibe, Rebitol, Ribasphue)
Interferon

Drugs for hepatitis A:
Havrix Hep A vaccine 1 ml IM

Immunoglobulin
Gamastan S/D (Immune Glob G)

Drugs for Hepatitis B:
Entecavir (Baraclude)
Tenofovir (Viread)
Tenofovir Alafenamide (Vemlidy)
Lamivudine (Epivir, Zeffix, Heptodin)
Adefovir (Hepsera)
Immunoglobulin
Interferon

Chapter 17

Hematological Disorders

Common hematological problems involving aging patients addressed in this book include anemia, lymphomas, multiple myeloma, bone marrow disorders, leukemia, and coagulopathies.

Anemia

Older adults present with anemia with nonspecific symptoms, complaining of loss of energy or strength. They may complain of dyspnea on exertion, tachycardia, fatigue, or palpitation. Severe cases may exhibit lightheadedness, orthostatic hypotension, or syncope.

It is estimated that over three million adults over age sixty-five have anemia. One-third have anemia of nutritional origin, one-third have anemia of inflammation, and the rest have an unknown cause.

Anemia of nutritional origin is due to poor intake of iron, vitamins, and folic acid. Anemia of inflammation is due to chronic illnesses such as infections, rheumatologic disorders, malignancies, and postsurgical changes in the gut. Anemia of unexplained origin in the older adult is due to low bone marrow activity with a low reticulocyte count. It may be myelodysplastic syndrome (MDS). Aging patients also have impaired erythropoietin response. Chronic blood loss from hemorrhoids or gastrointestinal malignancies or peptic ulcer disease is a condition that can lead to microcytic anemia. Hemolytic anemia can be intrinsic immune disorders or metabolic disorders or from extrinsic reasons, such as hemolytic substances or allergic reactions.

Treatment involves correction of nutritional deficiencies, administration of iron, vitamin B-12, folic acid, correction of underlying disorders that led to anemia, stoppage of blood loss, administration of erythropoietin stimulating agents such as Neupogen or Epogen, treatment of renal failure, consideration for intravenous iron or supplemental therapy, treatment of cancer conditions, and finally judicious administration of blood transfusion.

Leukemia

Chronic lymphocytic leukemia (CLL). CLL is the most prevalent form of leukemia in the older adult population. There is an accumulation of neoplastic B-lymphocytes in blood, bone marrow, liver, and spleen. Over half of these patients are asymptomatic and may end up living their natural course of life despite the presence of this bone marrow disorder. Hence treatment is started only if the patient becomes symptomatic with fever, night sweats, weight loss, and enlarged lymph nodes. In such cases, chemotherapy is recommended using chlorambucil or Fludarabine or Rituximab.

The Rai system is used to classify disease. A low-risk classification involves bone marrow and blood only. Intermediate risk involves lymph nodes with lymphadenopathy, lymphocytosis, and/or hepatomegaly or splenomegaly. A high-risk classification involves lymphocytosis, anemia, and thrombocytopenia.

Chronic myelogenous leukemia (CML). CML is a myeloproliferative disorder resulting from neoplastic transformation of myeloid elements. It can occur at any age, including older adults. Patients may present with fatigue, malaise, fever, anemia, thrombocytopenia, easy bruising, and splenomegaly. Tyrosine kinase inhibitors are used in the treatment of this condition.

Multiple myeloma (MM)

In patients with MM, there is a proliferation of plasma cells and plasma cell precursors. Initially there is loss of T-cell-mediated control of early B-cell development. Then there is accumulation of immunoglobulins and malignant transformations.

Patients complain of bone pain due to bone resorption. Resultant hypercalcemia leads to nausea, vomiting, constipation, fatigue, lethargy, and new onset diabetes mellitus. Half of patients develop renal failure due to light chain precipitation in renal tubules leading to obstruction and atrophy of nephrons. Amyloid and hyperviscosity cause retinopathy, congestive heart failure, mucosal bleeding, anemia, and neuropathy. A heightened risk for infections can result in mortality.

Diagnosis is with findings of 10 percent or more atypical plasma cells in bone marrow, monoclonal immunoglobulin in the serum, and light chain protein in the urine. X-rays of bones show osteolytic lesions, pathological fractures, and osteopenia.

Initial therapy is with melphalan and prednisone. Interferon helps to prolong remission. For resistant disease, one may choose vincristine, doxorubicin, and dexamethasone.

Plasmapheresis is performed to reduce hyperviscosity. Blood transfusion and erythropoietin are used to address anemia. Bisphosphonates are used to reduce hypercalcemia.

Coagulopathies

Older adults are prone to have coagulopathies with resultant easy bruising, hematoma formations, and intracranial bleeding or gastrointestinal bleeding for a variety of reasons. Age itself is a factor with weakened connective tissue, fibroblasts, and bone marrow.

Patients can be on various medications that result in thrombocytopenia. Certain medications such as aspirin Plavix affect the coagulation system. They can be on medications to prevent clot formation following pulmonary embolism or systemic embolism or deep vein thrombosis or following placement of metallic stents or valves in the cardiovascular system.

The patient is also prone to diseases of the liver, spleen, bone marrow or cancer conditions that increase the risk of excessive bleeding.

Chapter 18

Orthopedic and Rheumatologic Conditions

Arthritis occurs in old age, resulting in swollen painful joints. Patients have trouble walking, sitting, or balancing, resulting in a tendency to fall and fracture bones. Osteoporosis and osteoarthritis are part of the aging process. In addition, a variety of other arthritic conditions—such as rheumatoid arthritis, psoriatic arthritis, gout, and muscular dystrophies—can occur. The cartilage in the joints, such as the knee and shoulder, starts wearing down, causing pain. Back pain is common in older adults due to prolapsed intervertebral disc, fracture of the vertebrae, and cancer conditions.

Osteoporosis

Osteoporosis is demineralization of the bones, resulting in the matrix of bones becoming brittle. The bones break or crumble easily. Even minimal trauma can cause fractures of hip or long bones or fracture of vertebrae resulting in kyphosis. Ribs can fracture from coughing spells related to flu or bronchitis.

The most common causes of calcium loss from the bones are diabetes mellitus, estrogen deficiency in postmenopausal state in women, alcoholism, hyperparathyroidism, malabsorption, multiple myeloma, renal failure, and vitamin D deficiency.

Bone density tests and x-rays are useful tests. A key part in any evaluation is to identify any underlying diseases or primary malignancies that could contribute to bone loss.

Calcium replacement therapy can be through measures such as milk or fruits and calcium supplements. Vitamin D replacement and exposure to sunlight are beneficial. Exercises to strengthen long bones and prevention of falls have benefits as well. Bisphosphonates are antiresorptive agents that bind hydroxyapatite crystals on bone surfaces and inhibit osteoclast function. They have side effects but help to reduce the risk of bone fractures. Hormone replacement therapy has been controversial for years but is approved for postmenopausal women. Combined estrogen and progesterone therapy can increase bone density. Raloxifene is a selective estrogen receptor modulator that binds to and activates estrogen receptors. Calcitonin acts directly on osteoclasts with inhibitory effects on bone resorption but is only rarely used. Denosumab is a human monoclonal antibody that is found helpful in reducing osteoclastic function. Teriparatide is a synthetic parathyroid hormone that helps to remodel bones and reduces fractures. Prompt surgery to correct fractures and collapsed vertebrae will prevent further damage.

The latest recommendation is to plan medication sequencing in advance of initiation of therapy to maximize benefits. At this time, initiating treatment of a naïve patient with Teriparatide (PTH) followed by Denosumab seems to be the most effective approach.

Table 24

Medications for osteoporosis

Bisphosphonates:
Alendronate (Fosamax) 5 to 10 mg orally daily
Risedronate (Actonel) 5 mg orally daily
Ibandronate (Boniva) 2.5 mg orally daily
Zoledronic acid (Zometa) 4 mg IV every twelve months

Hormone replacement therapy:
Estrogen
Progesterone

Selective estrogen receptor modulator:
Raloxifene 60 mg orally daily
Calcitonin 200 IU nasal spray daily

Human monoclonal antibody:
Denosumab (Prolia) 60 mg subQ every six months

Synthetic Parathyroid hormone:
Teriparatide (Forteo) 20 mcg subQ daily for twenty-four months

---

Osteoarthritis (OA)

OA is the most common age-related arthritis involving major joints. The cartilage gets worn out. Cell proliferation occurs in and around the joint leading to swelling and pain. It can be from wear and tear of aging or repeated trauma, stress on the joint, obesity, postural changes, sporting activities, prior surgery, hemochromatosis, gout, Wilson's disease, or genetic factors.

It is a slowly progressive and insidious disorder, leading to increasing disability with pain, swelling, crepitus, contractures, difficulty in ambulation, sitting, or standing. There is thickening of the joint capsule, synovial hypertrophy and inflammation, meniscal degeneration, osteophyte formation, degradation and loss of articular cartilage, thickening of subchondral bone with bone marrow lesions, and bone cyst formation. Osteophytes form at the joint margins.

X-rays show loss of cartilage, loss of joint space, marginal osteophyte formation, and sclerosis of subchondral bone.

Treatment with medical measures includes NSAIDs, opioids, glucosamine sulfate, chondroitin sulfate, and Vitamin D. Physiotherapy with heat, non-weight bearing exercises, and muscle-strengthening exercises, swimming, and body weight loss programs are tried. Intra articular injections of Zilretta (triamcinolone acetonide) or hyaluronidase and platelet-rich plasma (PRP) are useful measures in relieving pain. Other measures tried orthotic devices, acupuncture, massage, TENS (transcutaneous electric nerve stimulation), and pulsed electromagnetic field stimulator (PEMF). Final stages require surgery. Procedures include arthroscopic lavages, realignment osteotomy, joint fusion (arthrodesis), or total joint replacements (arthroplasty).

Rheumatoid arthritis (RA)

RA is an autoimmune disorder that affects small joints, causing pain, swelling, deformity, nodule formation, and disability along with systemic symptoms of malaise, anorexia, and weight loss. These are caused by a humoral immune response with rheumatoid factor, IgM, IgG, or IgA.

In addition, there can be extra-articular manifestations such as anemia, eosinophilia, thrombocytosis, Felty's syndrome, neutropenia, lymphadenopathy, osteoporosis, splenomegaly, vasculitis, pericarditis, pleural effusion, Raynaud's phenomenon, interstitial fibrosis, keratoconjunctivitis, scleritis, corneal ulcerations, and amyloidosis.

Lab tests show elevated ESR and positive rheumatoid factor. X-rays show periarticular osteopenia, deformities, swellings, and symmetrical involvements.

Initial therapy includes aspirin and azathioprine and advanced to methotrexate or sulfasalazine. Steroid injections may be needed. Hydroxychloroquine, Enbrel, Arava, and Remicade are other medications. Physiotherapy, splints, hot soaks, swimming, or walking exercises are helpful.

Gout

Gout is due to hyperuricemia. It can be due to overproduction of urates or underexcretion of uric acid. Either way, it leads to saturation of extracellular body fluids with urates, leading to crystal formation and deposition of powdery white material in and around joints associated with inflammation, pain, and swelling, the features being called tophus/tophi formation. There can be attacks of acute arthritis of single joints or tophi formations near metatarsal joints. There is hyperuricemia in all cases. Risk of uric acid stone formation in the kidney is noted. Pseudogout is a condition where calcium pyrophosphate deposition occurs in large joints following trauma or surgery.

It is recommended that individuals with gout avoid high purine foods such as shellfish, wild game and meat products, and alcohol. Hydration is necessary. Treatment of acute gouty arthritis is with NSAIDs, indomethacin, and colchicine. Intra-articular injection of steroids is helpful when oral drugs are contraindicated. Allopurinol is used for chronic gout when overproduction of urates is suspected. It is a competitive inhibitor of xanthine oxidase. When underexcretion is suspected, uricosuric agents such as probenecid or sulfinpyrazone are used.

Back pain

Almost every adult experiences back pain some time or another, most of which are musculoskeletal in origin and are of short duration. Often these are because of falls, trauma, sporting injuries, excessive weight bearing, or muscle sprains.

However, older adults are more likely to suffer from chronic back pain. These are because of osteoporosis, fracture of vertebrae, kyphosis, spinal stenosis, prolapse of intervertebral disc with compression of the spinal nerve roots, or metastatic cancer deposits in the vertebrae and tuberculosis. Sudden excruciating low back pain followed by hypotension and shock is the hallmark of a ruptured abdominal aortic aneurysm.

One frequent problem is degeneration of the intervertebral disc, leading to compression of one vertebra over the next, seen as a loss of intervertebral space in X-rays along with laxity of the longitudinal ligaments and subluxation of facet joints. There is pain in the calf, leg, quads, and hip upon walking. Compression of the nerve roots can cause neurological changes with motor and sensory changes, muscle wasting, and back pain with radiation to the thigh. MRI is helpful in furthering the diagnosis. Initially, conservative therapies with rest and exercises and epidural steroid injections are offered. Surgery is an option if there is no improvement or if there is progressive neurological damage. This may be a discectomy, fusion, or decompression.

Upper limb musculoskeletal diseases

These problems include adhesive capsulitis of the shoulder, rotator cuff problems, biceps tendon problems, olecranon bursitis and tennis elbow, carpal tunnel syndrome, de Quervain's contracture, and scaphoid injury.

Adhesive capsulitis, commonly known as frozen shoulder, is idiopathic and may present as pain or contracture. There is excessive hyperplastic fibroplasia and collagen deposit in glenohumeral synovial joint and pericapsular tissues, resulting in adhesive contracture similar to Dupuytren's contracture in the palm. Genetic predisposition is considered in etiology even though it manifests more commonly in the fifth or sixth decades of life. Radiology imaging studies are done to rule out other pathologies, but the diagnosis of frozen shoulder is still a clinical one. Treatment is nonsurgical with physiotherapy, intra-articular injections of steroids or hyaluronidase, and pain medications. Often the disease is self-limiting.

Table 25

Non-narcotic medications of use for pain control
Acetaminophen (APAP) 650 mg q four to six hours
Aspirin (ASA) 650 mg q four to six hours
Excedrin (acetaminophen, aspirin, caffeine)
Nonacetylated salicylates:
Choline magnesium salicylate (Tricostal, Trisilate) 1,500 mg
 twice daily
Magnesium salicylate (Novasal) two tabs q six to eight hours
Salsalate 1,500 mg twice daily
Nonselective NSAIDS:
Diclofenac (Cataflam, Voltaren, Zipsor, Zorvolex) 50 to
150 mg/day in divided doses
Pennsaid solution 1.5 percent apply on knee q six hours
Enteric coated (Arthrotec) one tab q eight to twelve hours
Diflunisal (Dolobid) 500–1,000 mg/day in two doses
Etodolac (Lodine) 200–400 mg q six to eight hours
Fenoprofen (Nalfon) 200–600 mg q six to eight hours
Flurbiprofen (Ansaid) 200–300 mg/day in divided doses
Ibuprofen 1,200–3,200 mg/day in divided doses
Ketoprofen (Orudis) 50–75 mg q eight hours
Ketorolac (Toradol) 10 mg q four to six hours IM or IV
Meclofenamate sodium 200–400 mg/day in divided doses
Mefenamic acid (Ponstel) 250 mg q six hours *discontinued in US*
Meloxicam (Mobic) 7.5–15 mg/day
Nabumetone (Relafen) 500–1,000 mg q twelve hours
Naproxen (Naprosyn) 220–500 mg q twelve hours
Oxaprozin (Daypro) 1,200 mg/day
Piroxicam (Feldene)10 mg/day
Sulindac (Clinoril) 600–1,800/day in divided doses *discontinued in US*
Tolmetin (Tolectin) 600–1,800 mg/day in divided doses
Trolamine salicylate (Aspercreme) three to four per day 10
percent soln
Selective COX-2 inhibitor:
Celecoximab (Celebrex) 100–200 mg q twelve hours
Muscle relaxant:
Baclofen (Gablofen, Lioresal) 5–15 mg PO

Hip fractures

A hip fracture (fractured femur) is a significant injury with complications that can be life-threatening. Hip fracture risk increases with age.

The risk increases because bones weaken with age (osteoporosis). Multiple medications, poor vision, fragility, and balance problems predispose older adults to be more likely to fall—one of the most common causes of hip fractures.

A hip fracture almost always requires surgical repair or a replacement, followed by physical therapy. Taking steps to maintain bone density and avoid falls can help prevent a hip fracture. The consequence of a fall may lead to an inability to get up or walk, severe pain in the hip or groin, or an inability to put weight on the leg on the side of the injured hip. The patient or a medical professional might note bruising and swelling in and around the hip area, a shorter leg on the side of the injured hip, and an outward turning of the leg on the side of the injured hip.

In older adults, a hip fracture is most often a result of a fall from standing height. In people with very weak bones, a hip fracture can occur simply by standing on the leg and twisting, and thus the fracture precedes the fall.

Diminished bone density and muscle mass associated with age are risk factors for hip fractures. Older adults can also have problems with vision and balance, which can increase the risk of falling.

Hip fractures occur in women about three times more often than they do in men. Women lose bone density faster than men do, and this is in part because the drop in estrogen levels—which occurs with menopause—accelerates bone loss. However, men also can develop dangerously low levels of bone density.

Osteoporosis, the condition of weakened bones, is the most common risk factor, but other conditions that pose a risk are thyroid, intestinal, and neurologic problems. Lack of calcium and vitamin D in the diet of young people lowers peak bone mass and increases the risk of fractures later in life. It is also important to get enough calcium and vitamin D in older age to maintain bone density and overall strength. Underweight status also increases the risk of bone loss. Lack of regular weight-bearing exercise such as walking can result in weakened bones and muscles, making falls and fractures more likely.

Tobacco and alcohol both can interfere with the normal processes of bone building and maintenance, resulting in bone loss.

A hip fracture can reduce independence and sometimes shorten life. About half the people who have a hip fracture cannot regain the ability to live independently.

Hip fractures will limit mobility, and there is a considerable risk that complications can cause blood clots in the legs or lungs, bedsores, pneumonia, and a loss of muscle mass, increasing the risk of falls, injuries, and death. Depression is another negative effect of a fractured hip. Most people recover from the depression associated with a hip fracture in about a year as they return to normal activities.

Prevention is a key part in reducing hip fractures. The most important actions to address risks are the following:

- Getting enough calcium and vitamin D. Men and women aged fifty and older should consume 1,200 milligrams of calcium a day and 600 international units of vitamin D a day.
- Exercising to strengthen bones and improve balance. Weight-bearing exercises such as walking help support peak bone density. Exercise also increases overall strength, decreasing the risk of falling. Balance training is also important to reduce the risk of falls since balance deteriorates with age.
- Avoiding smoking or excessive drinking. Tobacco and alcohol use can reduce bone density. Drinking too much alcohol can also impair balance and increase the risk of falling.
- Assessing the home for hazards. Removing throw rugs, keeping electrical cords against the wall, and clearing excess furniture and anything else that could precipitate a fall and making sure all rooms and passageways are well lit are recommended.
- Checking vision. Get an eye exam every other year or more often, especially for those with diabetes or eye disease.
- Using an assistive device such as a cane, walking stick, or walker. If the individual is not steady when walking, a health-care provider or physical or occupational therapist would be of benefit and can reduce fall risk.

PMR/ temporal arteritis

Polymyalgia rheumatica (PMR) is a common chronic inflammatory condition of unknown etiology that affects older adults. Proximal myalgia of the hip and shoulder girdle characterizes it with accompanying morning stiffness that lasts for over one hour. Approximately 15 percent of patients with PMR develop giant cell arteritis (GCA), and 40–50 percent of patients with GCA have associated PMR. Despite the similarities of age at onset and the clinical manifestations, the relationship between GCA and PMR has not been clearly proven.

PMR is a clinical diagnosis based on the complexity of presenting symptoms and the exclusion of other potential diseases. Corticosteroids are considered the treatment of choice, and a rapid response to low-dose corticosteroids is considered pathognomonic. Dosages of five to ten milligrams of Prednisone can improve symptoms rapidly, but patients might need therapy for twelve to eighteen months. Patients who are at risk for relapse, have steroid-related adverse effects, or need prolonged steroid therapy may benefit from the addition of methotrexate or tocilizumab.

Patients have an excellent prognosis. Exacerbations may occur if steroids are tapered too rapidly, however, and relapse is also common.

Temporal arteritis

Giant cell arteritis (GCA), or temporal arteritis, is a systemic inflammatory vasculitis of unknown etiology that occurs in older adults and can cause a wide variety of systemic, neurologic, and ophthalmologic complications. GCA is the most common form of systemic vasculitis in adults. Other names for GCA include arteritis cranialis, Horton disease, granulomatous arteritis, and arteritis of the aged.

GCA is classified as a large-vessel vasculitis but typically also involves medium and small arteries, particularly the superficial temporal arteries—hence the term *temporal arteritis*. In addition, GCA most commonly affects the ophthalmic, occipital, vertebral, posterior ciliary and proximal vertebral arteries. Medium- and large-sized vessels that may be involved include the aorta and the carotid, subclavian, and iliac arteries. Histopathologically, GCA is marked by the transmural inflammation of the intima, media, and adventitia of affected arteries as well as patchy infiltration by lymphocytes, macrophages, and multinucleated giant cells. Mural hyperplasia can narrow the arterial lumen, resulting in distal ischemia.

Age and female sex are known risk factors for GCA. A genetic component seems likely, and infection may have a role.

Common signs and symptoms of GCA reflect the involvement of the temporal artery and other medium-sized arteries of the head and the neck and include visual disturbances, headaches, jaw claudication, neck pain, and scalp tenderness. Constitutional manifestations such as fatigue, malaise, and fever may also be present.

GCA should always be considered in the differential diagnosis of a new-onset headache in patients fifty years of age or older with an elevated erythrocyte sedimentation rate. Temporal artery biopsy is still the criterion standard for the diagnosis of this granulomatous vasculitis. However, increasing evidence supports the use of imaging studies for diagnosis in patients at high clinical risk.

Visual loss is one of the most significant causes of morbidity in GCA. Permanent visual impairment may occur in as many as 20 percent of patients, and in some cases, GCA can cause bilateral blindness. Acutely diagnosed GCA should be considered a true neuro-ophthalmic emergency.

Prompt initiation of treatment may prevent blindness and other potentially irreversible ischemic sequelae of GCA. Corticosteroids are the mainstay of therapy. In steroid-resistant cases, drugs such as tocilizumab, cyclosporine, azathioprine, or methotrexate are options as steroid-sparing agents. The typical patient with GCA remains on steroid therapy for two years.

Chapter 19

Surgery and Anesthesia in the Aging Population

The older adults are at higher risk for complications, morbidity, and mortality following surgery or anesthesia because of associated cardiorespiratory conditions or lower immune status and nutritional status. Their ability to fight the infections or survive trauma of surgery is lower than the youngsters. Hence careful planning and conduct of surgery is essential.

Very often, surgery can be avoided or downgraded to a lower magnitude procedure. For example, it is questionable to treat a ninety-plus-year-old patient in bedridden state with insertion of permanent pacemaker, defibrillators, chemotherapy, dialysis, and complex surgical procedures. Their life expectancy is minimal. Their quality of life is poor. They may have a Living Will and DNR instructions. It is important to discuss the pros and cons of life-prolonging procedures with family members and legal guardians.

Less invasive procedures are chosen in many instances. For example, an aortic aneurysm in an eighty-year-old is preferably treated by endovascular stent placement instead of open repair. A palpable cancer of the breast in a ninety-year-old can be managed with a lumpectomy alone to prevent local progression instead of a full cancer surgery such as modified radical mastectomy and chemotherapy. When possible, laparoscopic procedures may be better tolerated than open abdominal surgery. Prolonged surgery is best avoided in favor of short procedures.

Similarly, when choosing anesthesia, one may want to avoid general anesthesia with muscle relaxation and use shorter techniques, such as local anesthesia with sedation, use of ketamine or fentanyl, spinal anesthesia, or regional blocks. General anesthesia with intubation and prolonged muscle relaxation can lead to ventilator dependence postoperatively. The patient's coughing and deep breathing ability is compromised and can easily develop atelectasis and pneumonia.

Preoperative evaluation should include cardiac clearance for the intended procedure by a cardiologist. Emphasis is placed on stress tolerance since surgery and anesthesia is a major trauma to the body. Resting EKG, stress test on treadmill or by nuclear technology, and echocardiogram to evaluate valvular function and ejection fraction are options. Finally, it may be necessary to do a coronary angiogram and do procedures such as coronary angioplasty or stent placement to make them stable for surgery. Postoperatively, these patients need monitoring for various cardiac arrhythmias and congestive heart failure. Fluid and electrolyte management require close attention to avoid fluid overload or dehydration. These patients are at risk for developing silent heart attacks. Aortic stenosis should be identified and corrected, as necessary. Elective surgery may be delayed while awaiting a cardiac evaluation. Sometimes the patients are on anticoagulants for atrial fibrillation or prior medical problems such as deep vein thrombosis (DVT) or pulmonary embolism (PE). The coagulation profile needs to be corrected to undergo the surgery and anticoagulation can be restarted postoperatively. If the patient is taking antiplatelet medication, such as aspirin or Plavix, these medications need to be stopped at least five days prior to major surgery.

A pulmonary evaluation might include recommendations for cessation of smoking and the need for chest physiotherapy. Observe for evidence of COPD and the potential for long-term ventilator support postoperatively. Diabetes mellitus and glycemic control need attention intraoperatively and postoperatively. Renal status, urinary tract infection, need for indwelling catheter, electrolyte, and blood, gas, and fluid requirement are to be assessed.

Older patients have higher risk for dementia, withdrawal symptoms from alcohol and drugs, potential for postoperative delirium, psychological derangements, confusion, and falls. They may have difficulty in comprehension. It is important to have family members or guardians involved in all steps of treatment, from consent to disposition.

Table 26

List of narcotic medications for pain control

Morphine (Astramorph, Avinza, Kadian, MS contin, Oramorph SR, Kadian)
Hydromorphone (Dilaudid, Exalgo) 1 mg IV/IM, 5–10 mg PO
Demerol (Pethidine, Meperidine) 50–100 mg PO, IM, IV
Hydrocodone/acetaminophen (Vicodin, Lortab, Lorcet, Norco)
Hydrocodone (Hysinga, Zohydro ER)
Oxycodone (OxyContin, Oxecta, Roxicodone)
Oxycodone/acetaminophen (Percocet, Endocet, Roxicet)
Fentanyl (Actiq, Duragesic, Abstral, Onsolin, Fentora, Ionsys, Lazanda, Sublimaze, Subsys) 50–100 mcg slow IV over two minutes
Tramadol (Ultram) 100 mg PO six to eight hours

Acetaminophen/Tramadol (Ultracet) 325 mg, Acet/37.5 Tram Codeine

Acetaminophen with codeine (Tylenol no. 3 or no. 4) 300 mg / 15 mg, 300 mg / 30 mg, 300 mg / 60 mg

Hydrocodone bitartrate/ibuprofen (Reprexain)

Talwin (Pentazocine) 20–40 mg IM

Table 27

List of medications for sleep management

(To be used with caution in aged population)
Nembutal (Pentobarbital) 150–200 mg IM
Seconal (Phenobarbital) 15–100 mg PO/IM
Trazodone (Desyrel) 150 mg PO per day in divided doses
Benzodiazepines
Temazepam (Restoril) 15 mg PO/night
Triazolam (Halcion) 0.25 mg PO
Quazepam (Doral) 7.5 mg to 15 mg PO
Doxepin (Silenor) 6 mg PO
Eszopiclone (Lunesta) 1 mg PO
Lemborexant (Dayvigo) 5 mg PO
Ramelton (Rozerem) 8 mg PO
Suvorexant (Belsomra) 5–15 mg PO
Zaleplon (Sonata) 5–10 mg PO
Zolpidem (Ambien, Edluar, Intermezzo) 5 mg PO before sleep
Antihistamines
Melatonin

Chapter 20

Physical Therapy and Rehabilitation

Physical therapy and rehab measures are now integral parts of recovery from any type of major illness or surgery. After surgery, a period of recovery is desirable to get the best outcome. This recovery period is used to maximize the healing and return to normality. While all patients need this step toward healing, older patients have greater needs for assistance and encouragement. The word *physikos* means physical, and *iatreia* means art of healing (Greek origin), thus meaning healing by physical methods, such as application of heat, cold, massage, exercise, manipulation, and stretching. Physiatry as a medical specialty is the practice of physical therapy and rehabilitation.

Physiotherapy and rehabilitation are extensions of treatments for a multitude of medical problems. In systemic lupus erythematosus, there is muscle weakness and arthritis, predominantly involving hands and knees, and isometric exercises are recommended. In osteoarthritis, weight bearing joints are affected, and the goal is pain reduction and function optimization. Swimming and aerobic aquatic programs provide nonweight bearing activities. Tai chi gives stop-and-rest bursts of activities.

Cervical disc problems can be because of herniated nucleus pulposus, degenerative disc disease, or internal disc disruption. Of these, degenerative disc disruption (DDD) is often due to aging, poor nutrition, smoking, and atherosclerosis. Other contributors to DDD are heavy lifting, trauma, whiplash, prolonged sedentary work, and repetitive stress. MRI is the best test to evaluate the problem. Other studies include plain x-ray of the neck, nerve conduction studies, and EMG (electromyogram). Initial treatment involves stabilization exercises, postural training, cervical traction, and steroid injections. Surgery is appropriate if there is a neurogenic bowel or bladder problem or if there is a worsening neurological deficit. This may involve cervical arthroplasty or fusion.

Upper-extremity musculoskeletal problems can be treated by nonsurgical treatment involving physiotherapy. Frozen shoulder syndrome, biceps tendon rupture, or biceps tendinitis is treated with rest, soft immobilization, cold compression with ice or cold packs, NSAIDS, and non-weight bearing exercises. Initial treatment of carpal tunnel syndrome can include splints and rest to the wrist. Rotator cuff injuries in the early phase can be effectively treated by physiotherapy with rest to shoulder and careful exercise regimen. In addition, ultrasound therapy, pulsed electromagnetic field therapy, thermotherapy, and TENS treatments are found useful.

Physiotherapy is useful in the treatment of RSD (reflex sympathetic dystrophy), or complex regional pain syndrome (CRPS) referred to as causalgia in the past. There is disproportionate extremity pain and swelling with sympathetic and motor symptoms. It would be necessary to start therapy at low threshold levels and make progressive increases; starting a program with non-weight bearing and then advancing to slow increases in weight bearing. Gradual desensitization to sensory stimuli is done.

Preventive
Health Care
for the Older Adult

Chapter 21

Dietary Recommendations and Nutritional Requirements

The fourth-century BC Greek physician Hippocrates said, "Let food be your medicine." We can consider food as a medicine for many illnesses. It was true in the fourth-century BC, and it is still true today.

The amount of food consumed, number of calories consumed, type of food, getting necessary components such as vitamins, minerals, and proteins, type of drinks and calories, and avoiding harmful food items are a range of factors to be considered for supporting good health as we age.

Type of food. A Mediterranean diet is considered one of the best examples of a good diet. It includes vegetables, lentils, beans, nuts, fruits, fish or fish oil supplements, and olive oil. It is best to avoid fatty food, sugary stuff, Cola drinks, animal fat, and red meat.

Unhealthy diets consist of red meat items such as barbecued beef and hamburgers and cheeseburgers, French fries and doughnuts, pastries and cakes, potato chips, and Cola drinks. Type 2 diabetes can be controlled with diet by reducing carbohydrates such as rice, bread, sugars, and sweets and by use of medications.

A randomized clinical trial of 48,000 women conducted by Women's Health Initiative in 2019 confirmed that postmenopausal women have reduced risk of dying from breast cancer if they followed a low-fat diet with fruits, vegetables, and grains compared to those who had high-fat diet with nonvegetarian food.

Similarly, dietary control has been shown to be effective against hypertension, heart diseases, stroke, diabetes mellitus, and other types of cancers such as pancreatic, gastric, colorectal, and hepatic and such visceral malignancies in prior studies.

Reduce salt. Avoiding excess salt is a good measure in reducing heart attacks, reducing clogged arteries, and improving kidney function. Dr. Surender Reddy Neravetla has published *Salt Kills* and addresses the adverse effects of excess salt in daily food. He recommends removal of salt and pepper shakers from dining tables altogether.

Quality. Omega-3 fatty acids have favorable effects on blood pressure and plaque buildup inside arteries.

Omega-3 fatty acids are found in fish or fish oil. For those who consume a vegetarian diet, this supplement can is available in a pill form. Antioxidants can fight to slow growth of cancer and increase longevity of cells. They have antiaging properties when one considers oxidation as a cause of cell death. Antioxidants are found in blueberries, strawberries, and fresh fruits. Glucosinolates convert to compounds that slow growth of cancer cells. They are found in broccoli and other green vegetables. Nuts and seeds can repair chromosomes, enhancing cellular longevity. Polyphenols found in apples can retard the growth of cancer cells. Berries increase memory power and delay the onset of dementia. Cranberry juice, pomegranate juice, and red wine have resveratrol, which has been proposed to reduce heart attacks and cholesterol plaque accumulation inside arteries.

Antioxidants. Cellular metabolism causes oxidation, which leads to formation of free radicals. Excess accumulation of free radicals causes cell deterioration and eventual cell death. Antioxidants reduce free radical formation and thus prolong cell life. Antioxidants have a favorable impact by reducing illnesses and improving health. Antioxidants are found in many of the food items that cover the colors of the rainbow. Fresh fruits of all types, berries such as blueberry, strawberry, and raspberry and vegetables such as carrots, sweet potatoes, beets, and beans, green vegetables such as broccoli, cabbage, and spinach, pecan nuts, red tomatoes, red cabbage, and eggplants and turmeric have high concentrations of antioxidants. In summary, eating more fresh vegetables, fresh fruits, and nuts will provide antioxidants that will improve our health.

Fiber. There are benefits to having fiber in our diet because it provides volume in the stomach and has little, or no sugar compared to refined carbohydrates. Fiber allows food to be digested slowly with fewer fluctuations in sugar level in the blood. Fiber also allows one to eat fewer calories compared to items such as doughnuts and pastries. It reduces constipation and straining by adding bulk to stool. Diverticular disease of the colon is prevalent in Western countries and less common in Asian countries. One reason considered is the high-fiber diet consumed by the Asian population.

Supplements. One must focus on getting all the various minerals, vitamins, proteins, and essential fatty acids along with carbohydrates when planning a diet. Ancient Indian food items that include turmeric, ginger, and spices are combined to make sauces healthy.

Citrus fruits have vitamin C. Spinach has iron, and fresh fruits have other vitamins.

Quantity. Quantity of food intake needs control to avoid obesity. One method is to stop eating once the stomach is three quarters full, avoiding that last serving. Slowly, the stomach size shrinks, and the quantity of food can slowly be reduced. Another method is referred to as partial fasting, intermittent fasting, or timed meals. This method is to time or delay the first meal of the day for an extra few hours before starting a feeding cycle. Initially, the stomach will feel empty, and one can drink water. Slowly, the time interval between food intake is increased from six to eight hours and then eventually fourteen to sixteen hours, and the craving for food subsides. Another way to reduce the quantity of food is to eat slowly and in smaller amounts of food in each mouthful. Chew the food as long as possible, savor the taste, and take time to swallow before the next bite of food is consumed. Slow eating reduces total intake. Do not hurry and swallow big chunks and massive quantities. One refers to this as mindful eating, enjoying the taste.

Calories. Calorie count monitoring to avoid excessive calories per day. One way to reduce calories is to eat green leafy vegetables and other vegetables that are filling as opposed to sugary food and excess carbohydrates. Fruits and nuts are better used as snacks instead of bread, candies, muffins, and doughnuts. Water or unsweetened fruit juices can be consumed instead of Cola drinks or sugary drinks. Avoid sugary desserts such as ice cream, puddings, and cakes and instead have fresh fruits or skip the dessert altogether.

Other unhealthy diet items. Unhealthy foods eaten today are hazardous due to ultra processing of ingredients in manufacturing plants. In addition, this process alters the structure of fats. This processing converts them to trans fats, which are more likely to contribute to atherosclerosis. Examples of food items which are high in trans fats include animal fats, margarine, shortening, butter, ghee, fried foods, cakes, and cookies. More healthy substitutes/alternatives include olive oil, corn oil, sunflower oil, and fish oil. An individual's total fat intake needs to be considered.

Dietary recommendations for special needs.

Further detailed discussions are included in the chapters of the following disorders.

Diabetes mellitus: the goal is to reduce sugar while maintaining adequate calories and nutritional supplements.

Cardiovascular conditions: reduction of salt content, reduction of red meat, increase intake of omega-3 fatty acids such as fish or fish oil, and small quantities of red wine or cranberry juice are in consideration.

Renal conditions: hydrate well. Avoid high oxalate foods.

Hepatobiliary pancreatic problems: low-fat diet, no alcohol.

Osteoporosis, arthritis: high calcium, vitamin D, vitamin C, milk, and fish oil.

Swallowing and chewing problems: pureed food, liquid diet, enteral nutrition formula, and tube-feeding formula.

Anemia, cancer conditions: high-calorie, high-protein diet; iron-containing diet; spinach; and broccoli.

Thyroid problems: iodine-containing food, spinach.

Heartburn, acid reflux, peptic ulcer: bland diet, no spice, small meals, milk, and no alcohol.

Dementia: blueberries, strawberries, nuts, and seeds—high in protein and fat, low in sugar and carbohydrates.

Obesity prevention.

Obesity is a proven health hazard, which leads to a variety of medical problems and hastens death. It causes early onset of diabetes mellitus, osteoporosis, lung problems, heart problems, skin ulcerations, and eventually can reduce life expectancy by thirty years. Initial emphasis is on dietary control. Various dietary regimens or lifestyles are available. It is important to lose weight slowly with attention to vitamins, trace elements, and essential amino acids and essential fatty acids.

Overweight treatment.

Overweight and obesity are on the rise globally, with projections showing that by 2030, they could affect **half** of the population in industrialized countries. This alarming trend has led to a significant shift in perspective. Recognizing obesity as a complex medical condition, researchers and healthcare professionals are increasingly accepting the use of medication as a valuable tool for weight management.

The introduction of Glucagon-like Peptide-1 (GLP-1) receptor agonists has been a major turning point. These medications, including established options like Semaglutide (brand names: Ozempic, Wegovy) and newer entries like Tirzepatide (brand name: Mounjaro/Zepbound) and Liraglutide (brand name: Saxenda), are finding wider acceptance for their role in supporting weight management efforts.

Injectable noninsulin agents

GLP 1 receptor agonists:

Dulaglutide (Trulicity) 0.75–1.5 mg SubQ once a week

Exenatide extended release (Bydureon) 2 mg SubQ once a week

Liraglutide (Victoza) 0.6–1.8 mg SubQ once a day

Semaglutide (Ozempic, Rybelsus) 0.25 mg, 0.5 mg, 1 mg weekly

Tirzepatide (Mounjaro, Zepbound) 5mg, 10mg, 15mg weekly

Chapter 22

Exercise and Activities

Regular exercise of any type is immensely helpful to improve longevity and quality of life of older individuals. Exercises keep the body fit and trim, reduce weight, reduce the potential for obesity, maintain lower blood pressure, and reduce the risk for atherosclerosis and cancer. Increased physical activity reduces mortality rate and prolongs the quality of life. It improves muscle strength, joint flexibility, and bone density. It improves balance, coordination, and functionality. Physical activity and exercise reduce falls and fall-related injuries. It reduces the chance for osteoporosis, diabetes mellitus, and decreases cancers of the colon and breast. Social interaction is enhanced, and there is an improvement in a general sense of well-being and reduction in psychological problems. Mobility and independence improve. It also helps to improve sleep patterns. Endorphin, which is a happiness hormone, flows during exercises and keeps a person in a comfortable state called the zone. This allows peace and stress reduction, thus prolonging life and ensuring a healthier life. Exercise not only improves physical fitness. It also improves brain power.

Any form of physical activity qualifies, such as simple walking, swimming, bike riding, and running or workout in the gymnasium. Other activities would include taking part in one of the sporting activities such as tennis, golf, basketball, soccer, or hockey. Stretching exercises such as yoga, karate, tai chi, or pull-ups and push-ups are satisfactory. One must have a routine built into daily or weekly schedules. Dancing, skiing, or figure skating can be fun combined with music.

Exercise does not always mean sweaty, puffing, and straining strenuous activity. New guidelines suggest that less obvious movements can be considered exercise. Such activities include climbing the stairs instead of taking the elevator, raking the leaves, mowing the lawn, cleaning the patio, walking short distances at the workplace, shopping at the grocery store, cleaning the house, dancing, gardening, and bicycling for short distances instead of driving the car and so forth. Every movement counts, such as standing, walking while making phone calls, and standing on the subway or bus. These light activities are called NEAT (non-exercise activity thermogenesis) and can become supplementary to more vigorous activities for at least an hour or two per week. The new slogan is "Move more, sit less."

For aging adults, it may be difficult to participate in competitive sports. The easier activities include walking, stretching, and swimming. Window-shopping in the mall or visiting a park or zoo is a slow walking activity. Having a companion or family member to walk with the person adds to the enjoyment of the activity. Playing with children or grandchildren can be fun, bonding, and exercise. Unfortunately, only 10 percent of older people take part in regular activities lasting for thirty minutes or more.

Those who are frail or who have disabilities or chronic medical problems and heart disease should have a medical consultation and supervision before starting any new exercise programs. One may start with simple walking for short distances. Stretching or stationary bikes that do not require ambulation may be considered. Sitting down and up, slow muscle strengthening with light weights for those with muscle weakness, or aquatic programs for those with arthritic conditions are useful considerations. Physiotherapy and rehabilitation support is available for those recovering from illness such as heart attack, stroke, or trauma.

Chapter 23

Stress Reduction and Spirituality

Stress in life can reduce lifespan. Blood pressure and heart rate increase, which increases the potential for heart attacks and strokes. Judgment becomes impaired, resulting in dangerous actions and consequences, such as road rage, accidents, gun violence, and injuries. Stress also leads to obesity, alcohol use, or abuse of dependence on other chemical substances. Stress and its downstream consequences affect sleep patterns and work performance. It can affect marital life and social life and create family problems.

What causes stress in life? Very often it is from family issues, friction between expectations and reality.

Stress can manifest because of the following:

- A struggle between personalities, difficulty in adjusting and adapting between two or more people.
- A disappointment waiting to be expressed.
- A desire to be dominant or a refusal to be subservient.
- A question of what one wants versus what is available.
- A feeling of being trapped with no escape.
- Being in a frightening dark corner because of self-inflicted wounds.
- The inability to meet others' expectations, being diminished in honor or respect.
- A difficulty in expressing one's thoughts and needs because of constraints in the society and family structure.
- A choking sensation due to the dominant stature or pressure from parents or peers.
- A failure in performance at school or at the workplace.
- A physical disfigurement or complex that develops and becomes an issue caused by comments by others.
- Unresolved issucs from childhood developing into behavior patterns.
- Sexual abuse in childhood leaves indelible marks on the person's personality and outlook.
- Demands to take care of children or older adults with necessity to work along with demands at the workplace and associated transportation problems.

- Household issues can create stress and a burden.
- Divorces, abortions, murders, and suicides are different manifestations.
- Very often it is from family issues, friction between expectations and reality.

Chronic and acute illnesses can cause stress. Painful conditions such as

- arthritis, back pain, cancer problems, degenerative conditions,
- hearing and visual deficits,
- neurological problems such as paraplegia, paralysis, and incontinence,
- need for frequent visits to doctors and hospitals, and
- need for taking multiple medications

Another cause of stress is work related:

- Overwork, verbal abuse, disinterest in the type of work.
- Work that does not engage you or interest you.
- Working below your level of skill or working at a level above your ability.
- Need to have a better salary.
- Financial concerns.
- Need to move up to a higher level.
- Sexual harassment at work.
- Passing your turn for promotion, favoritism, nepotism, cronyism.
- Need for time off, need for vacation, or need to take care of children.
- Family responsibilities, inability to participate in family functions, nagging, bullying, harassment, sleeplessness, traffic, communication issues, transportation issues.
- Malpractice concerns.
- Undue expectations from clients, patients, or superiors.
- Constant interruptions.
- Need for high focus.
- Need for multitasking.
- Need for emergency actions on a regular basis.
- 24-7 involvement.
- Media attention.
- Social media.

Certain jobs such as that of a medical professional or air traffic controller are known to be high-stress jobs by the nature of work involved.

Work-related stress is expensive for both employer and employee. According to a report from the Center for Disease Control and Prevention in 2016, stress is the leading health problem in the workplace, affecting all levels of employees, leading to absenteeism, loss of productivity, and worker turnover. It also leads to depression, development of unhealthy habits including chemical dependency, and obesity. Measures found useful for reducing stress include regular work hours, adequate time off, greater autonomy, merit-based appreciation and growth opportunities, and economic security.

Irrespective of the cause of stress, it takes a toll on a person's health. The individual has diminished ability for performance and function. They withdraw from social and sporting activities. They tend to overeat and become obese. Lack of activity and obesity can lead to osteoporosis, hypertension, diabetes mellitus, stroke, and venous disorders. They also tend to be prone to develop behavioral problems, including commitment of suicides and homicides. The aftereffects lead to more stress as a vicious cycle.

Spirituality is the ability to accept our place and duty in this cosmic world. We can combine it with religious beliefs or places of worship, which could be a church, mosque, or a temple. However, to understand God, destiny, or fate, people benefit from the prop of a religion or a temple of worship or a priestly figure. But there are others who do not need such help. A higher power is the same in all religions. Prayer to a higher power calms the mind by agreeing to let the superior power remain in charge and in control of human lives. It helps to pray in times of distress and misfortune to find solace and comfort instead of feeling guilty and stressed. Certainly, most people will find peace and comfort in their last few days by placing themselves in the hands of God.

Stress, anxiety, and isolation can herald the onset of mental depression and inaction. Having a family, social activities, friends, group activities of any kind, exercise, visiting places of worship, meditation, and yoga are useful methods to address stress. One will have to analyze their own reasons for stress and write them down. This will help to overcome the stress points.

As noted above, scientific evidence shows that stress is harmful to health. Heart rate goes up, blood pressure goes up, and breathing becomes rapid and labored. The whole body, internally and externally, gets tensed up with increased adrenaline flow. Behavioral changes occur with anger and irritation, leading to verbal or physical reactions. There is an increased risk of heart attack and stroke. The digestive system shuts down with episodes of nausea or vomiting. Mental faculty is affected, causing errors, memory loss, and inability to focus, and job performance suffers. Headaches, asthma, hysteria, temper tantrums, work delinquencies occur. Stress affects social and physical wellness.

It is beneficial to incorporate relaxation techniques to reduce stress. Take a break for a few minutes when tired. Walk or talk. Have a cup of coffee or tea. Take a deep breath and do deep breathing exercises or stretching exercises. Take a power nap. It will do wonders. Meditation and yoga are other methods that help.

Unaddressed stress can lead to depression. One should seek medical advice. One may need counseling or medications. If left uncorrected, it can lead to further mental disorders or suicides.

Chapter 24

Medical Benefits of Yoga

Yoga has become more recognized as a meaningful preventative health-care measure all over the world. The United Nations proclaimed June 21 as International Yoga Day. In India, the day is met with great fanfare.

There is a fair amount of confusion, vagueness, and misunderstanding about yoga, especially on items relating to Ayurveda and associated historic, religious, and socioeconomic aspects.

When we focus on yoga, we recognize three main medical components: breathing exercises, stretching exercises, and meditation practices.

Breathing exercises

Breathing is part of life. We breathe regularly without even knowing that we are breathing. So how can it become an exercise?

We can voluntarily regulate breathing as a useful tool for achieving a relaxed state and a relaxed mind along with certain physical benefits. When one takes a deep breath slowly, holds it for a few seconds, and exhales slowly, several things happen. Automatically, our posture becomes more erect, and the chest, abdominal, and diaphragmatic muscles are engaged. This activity strengthens those muscles and enables one to cough and clear the respiratory passages better, helping to prevent bronchitis and pneumonia and faster recovery from common ailments and flu.

All the breathing passages cleanse, all the alveoli open, and fresh oxygen is delivered.

The mind becomes clearer and more relaxed. All the soft tissues and sphincter muscles relax.

Physiology of sinus arrhythmia is that the heart rate varies during breathing cycles. It is well-documented that one can reduce the heart rate by ten to twenty beats per minute by doing breathing exercises. Taking rapid breaths of short duration for   times leads to a feeling of reinvigoration and increased energy. This is because of the effects of hyperventilation, leading to mild respiratory alkalosis and hypocalcemia.

Breathing exercises help in the treatment of bronchial asthma, COPD (chronic obstructive pulmonary disease), congestive heart failure, sinusitis, and allergic rhinitis.

Singers, musicians, swimmers, and other athletes practice breath holding. It helps them to perform better. Athletes take a deep breath before they start a burst of activity, such as swimming, running, or wrestling.

Breathing exercise helps to relax and aids in stress reduction and anger management. Anxiety is reduced, muscle tension is relieved, and slouching and sagging shoulders are straightened.

Stretching exercises

Stretching is the part of yoga that gets the most attention in the media and in practice. Yoga is the practice of stretching various joints and ligaments and maintaining balance. Different postures and positions are described, touting various special benefits. The bulk of what is being offered as yoga includes doing various postures. These exercises allow flexibility of joints and tendons and improve muscle tone. They improve balancing ability, thus reducing falls and slips and reducing the chance for injuries.

Reduction in back pain, arthritis, fatigue syndrome, pain syndrome, migraine, and headaches are noted. There are reports of improved sleeping and sexual activity.

Most athletes engage in a period of stretching exercise before the actual commencement of their favorite sport. This allows them to perform better with an energy boost and loosened muscles and joints.

Stretching can be an exercise by itself, and it can be done not only in yoga but also in martial arts such as karate or tae kwon do and in other gymnastics. Passive static exercises of muscles are as good as active bursts of energy.

All exercises in any form help control blood pressure, weight, and diabetes mellitus and reduce the incidence of heart attacks, strokes, and cancers.

Meditation

Meditation is focused and controlled relaxation of the mind while keeping a sharp awareness for short periods of time. It requires a certain amount of practice initially; it is not the same as taking a nap. It is a timeout for the brain and is a voluntarily achieved state between conscious and subconscious mind. The connection between mind and body is well-documented, helping to control stress related conditions.

Meditation increases productivity, replenishes attention, solidifies memory power, and encourages creativity. It produces a state of relaxation, peace of mind, and a sense of tranquility.

Research with fMRI (functional MRI) shows that meditation can increase blood flow to the hippocampus and frontal areas of the brain and increase gray matter. EEG studies show increased alpha and theta activities in the frontal lobe. The amygdala, which is an area that processes emotional stimuli, shows decreased activity during meditation. This allows one to face uncomfortable situations with calmness and enables one to tolerate pain with fewer medications.

The net result is that there is stress reduction, increased empathy, happiness, and peacefulness. There is increased compliance with medical advice, reduction in drug dependence and alcohol abuse. There is less impulsive behavior leading to a reduction in gun violence, family quarrels, road rage, crimes, and accidents.

Meditation is very inexpensive, simple, and a possibility anywhere anytime and does not need any special equipment or setup. It is up to each person to effectively meditate by any method. Meditation can be combined with religious protocols or prayer, or it can be practiced by anyone regardless of spiritual beliefs.

It helps with management of anxiety disorders, diabetes, and hypertension, asthma, cancers, depression, and sleep disorders. It reduces dementia and the need for pain medications. Management of pain-related conditions and end-of-life issues are made easier. It also improves the immune activity of the body.

We can practice meditation in diverse ways. It can be focused or unfocused. One can repeat a certain syllable or prayer or a word or mantra. One can focus on a certain image or idol. It can also allow the mind to float free. We can combine it with chanting, or it can be total silence.

Combination of the above three steps

Medical benefits of yoga are well accepted and proven. Breathing, stretching, and meditation can be performed anywhere and at no expense. They improve both mental and physical well-being.

Yoga, breathing, and meditation practices can be tailored to a personal level. Group activities provide enjoyment and opportunity for socialization. Doing yoga in naturally scenic settings allows one to enjoy nature as yoga blends with appreciation of nature.

In 2009, the Nobel Prize was awarded for discovery of a telomerase enzyme that helps support the DNA structure of chromosomes longer, thus preventing aging of cells. Yoga and meditation are shown to increase the telomerase enzyme level, thus indirectly suggesting that one can prolong life and slow the aging process.

Yoga by itself does not cure any illnesses, but it works well as a complementary medical measure for better recovery from illnesses and to prevent illnesses related to lifestyle issues.

Over half of the medical problems and health-care expenses can be traced to societal problems, lifestyle issues, and behavioral problems as their root cause. We need to find methods that provide both mental and physical well-being. Yoga can be one such useful tool.

Chapter 25

Prevention of Cancer

Early detection of cancer offers patients the best potential for a cure. Screening and early detection is a well-established means for improved outcomes for breast cancers, colorectal cancers, and skin cancers. Cancers can be prevented by taking precautionary measures. For example, colonoscopy and removal of polyps can reduce incidence of colorectal cancers; use of sunscreens and avoiding sun exposure can reduce the risk of melanoma. Lifestyle habits such as diet, exercise, and avoidance of alcohol or smoking can reduce various malignancies. Screening for cancer and having regular medical checkups are good health measures.

Medicare and private medical insurance have evolved over the years such that currently they highly incentivize screening for preventable or curable diseases.

Skin. Early diagnosis of melanoma and squamous cell cancers can lead to curative treatments by simple wide, local excisions. Once skin cancers are advanced, cure rates are reduced even with complex therapies. Patients and physicians are advised to have any and every abnormal-looking skin lesion examined, biopsied, or excised if necessary.

Protecting against sun exposure is a useful measure. One may avoid direct exposure to the sun, apply sunscreen lotion, or cover up the body with clothing and head covering when outside.

Breast. Early diagnosis gives an almost 90 percent chance for a permanent cure. Routine physical examination, self-examination, and screening mammograms are satisfactory tools. Those who have a family history of breast cancers or who had prior gynecological cancers are at a higher risk. Gene testing for BRCA gene mutations is recommended for those at elevated risk.

In the April 30, 2024, issue of JAMA, the USPSTF (United States Preventive Services Task Force) published their latest recommendations for screening for breast cancers. The American Cancer Society (ACS) endorsed this recommendation that all women who are completely healthy with no risk factors get a routine mammogram every alternate year starting at age 40 until age 74. Those who have an elevated risk for cancer should start screening even much earlier or continue to further older age or get it done annually instead of biannually.

Cervix. Recommendations for cervical cancer screening include a

Pap smear (Pap test) between ages of 21 to 65 once every 3 years. In addition, those in age 30- 65 can optionally get a co-test for HPV (Human Papillomavirus) infection once every 5 years. According to a recent study published, there is a 90% reduction in cancer of cervix by doing routine both Pap smear and routine HPV vaccination. Cervical cancer is now considered a preventable cancer in the US. The only HPV vaccine available in the US is Gardasil 9 by Merck.

Routine HPV vaccination of all children (boys and girls) by age 11-12 is a recommendation to prevent not only cervical cancer but also oral and anal cancers, many are hesitant to follow this recommendation.

Lung. Avoid smoking at all costs. Also, avoid pollution, if possible, whether it is work related or environment related. Those who had exposure to asbestos and mining are at higher risk.

The USPSTF made specific recommendations for screening for lung cancer in March 2021. The screening is recommended only for adults between 50 and 80 years of age, who have a 20 pack-year history of smoking or are currently smoking or who quit smoking within the past 15-year period. The recommendation is low dose computed tomography of chest (LDCT) once a year. If the individual stopped smoking for more than 15 years or if they have serious other life-limiting conditions, then the screening is unnecessary. The recommended test is a CAT scan of the lungs with low radiation to detect tumors or other abnormalities in the lung fields. A pack year of smoking means smoking one pack of cigarettes per day for one year. Smoking includes cigarettes and cigars. The risk of vaping has not been confirmed.
Contact a physician for a physical examination and tests upon noticing coughing spells or hemoptysis.

Colorectal. Report any change in bowel habits or rectal bleeding for further evaluation.
With the observation of earlier onset of colorectal cancers, in 2022, the USPSTF and American Cancer Society recommended screening for colorectal cancers to start at age 45. Initial tests could be fecal occult blood test (FOBT) or DNA stool test (Cologuard) or fecal immunochemical test (FIT) once every 3 years. The FDA has approved a new RNA based test on the stool (Colo Sense).

Recommendations also include a colonoscopy once every 10 years until age 75. A virtual colonoscopy or sigmoidoscopy every 5 years is also an option. If any of the tests are abnormal, or if the person is at elevated risk or symptomatic, other investigations are appropriate.

Polyps diagnosed early can be removed endoscopically, thus preventing cancer formation.

Prostate. A routine PSA (prostate-specific antigen) has been met with controversy.

The American Cancer Society (ACS) recommends that all men above age 50 should get a blood test known as PSA (Prostate-Specific Antigen). A result of 4.0 ng/L or higher is the cutoff. Anything above this level would warrant additional evaluations and close follow-up. Otherwise, the test is to be repeated every other year. Progressively rising PSA level is of concern and warrants an evaluation by a urologist to rule out prostate cancer. Screening tests after the age of 80 or if life expectancy is less than 10 years for the individual may be unnecessary.

Lumps and bumps. All abnormal lumps and bumps should be evaluated. These lesions could be enlarged lymph nodes, which could be spread from another source or a primary lymphoma.

Testicular. Routine physical examinations should include palpation of testes for tumors, hydrocele, and hernia. Patients are also to report any abnormalities.

Visceral malignancies. One must follow up on unexplained weight loss, loss of appetite, vomiting, abdominal pain, or vomiting blood. A thorough physical examination and testing which might include a CT scan or GI endoscopy.

Brain tumors. One must not ignore unusual headaches, visual or hearing disturbances, falls, blackouts, fainting spells, or balancing problems. Consult a neurologist and get a CT scan or MRI of the brain.

Blood test. A regular complete blood count with peripheral smear can reveal leukemia, anemia, and bone marrow abnormalities. Certain markers for cancers such as CRP, alpha-fetoproteins, Ca-19, and Ca-125 have been described but are not specific for a diagnosis. Newer efforts to find a genetic abnormality for cancer are being investigated.

Other steps. Exercise regularly, eat a healthy diet, avoid dependence on alcohol and other chemical substances including smoking, and live in a healthy neighborhood.

A routine physical examination by a primary care physician and routine tests to evaluate any unusual symptoms might be a consideration during a yearly health maintenance exam.

A family history of cancers, history of previous cancers, history of exposure to cancerogenic agents, living in neighborhoods with pollutants, and working in radiology- or nuclear-related fields are conditions that should raise the level of alert and caution

Chapter 26

Other Preventive Health Care Measures

Mental tasks

Keeping the brain engaged will reduce the onset of dementia and will help support and grow new neuronal cells/connections. Mental work can be in different forms, such as playing board games, reading, writing, teaching, arts and crafts, chess, crossword puzzle, sudoku, and working. Simply reading a daily newspaper keeps one in touch with the local and national events, improves vocabulary, and keeps the brain engaged. Join a book club and discuss a book that you recently read. New neurons sprout by keeping the brain active by thinking, learning, and challenging it regularly. Functional MRI scans have shown increased gray matter and increased activity in the brain on those who challenge their minds at least two hours each day.

Sex

Touching is one of the five senses. The other senses are taste, smell, vision, and hearing. Eating delicious food, listening to pleasant music, seeing nature and beauty, and smelling a pleasant aroma brings peace and happiness. Touching, cuddling, and enjoyable sex also enhances connectedness, happiness, contentment and meaning in life, and improve social interaction and friendship. Oxytocin hormone is a happy hormone and is associated with normal biology of pregnancy and childbearing. A baby wants to be held, and it stops crying and smiles when it is held. So do the adults. Kissing, holding hands, feeling each other may or may not lead to sex, but it is certainly one of the wellness measures that improve good health both mentally and physically. Married people live longer and healthier than singles.

Sleep

Sleep requirements can vary, but on average, one should get seven to eight hours of sleep each night. It is enviable to sleep well, which provides much-needed rest to the body and mind. It is very refreshing for activities the following day. The human brain needs time off as it is part of the biorhythm. Older adults cannot sleep as soundly as younger individuals. Inadequate sleep leads to a variety of medical problems, including acceleration of the aging process. Insomnia is a medical problem for a sizable portion of the aging population. Having regular hours of sleep as a habit is most desirable. Watching less television, eating lighter meals, reading a book are methods to induce sleep. During sleep, the body and brain regenerate, repair, and replace damaged cells. Growth hormones are secreted during sleep, allowing younger individuals to grow while asleep. The immune system gets recharged. Melatonin is secreted, and neurons get time to rest and regenerate. Sleep deprivation causes various physical and mental problems, starting from irritability to instability and irrationality to unconsciousness. Unexplained weight gain is another consequence of sleep deprivation. About 20 percent of all road accidents are related to tiredness and sleeping while driving. Other side effects of inadequate sleep are confusion, memory loss, poor concentration, mood changes, clumsiness, frequent sicknesses, high blood pressure, type 2 diabetes mellitus, weight gain, low sex drive, infertility, heart disease, injuries, low athletic performance, short temper, higher chance of stroke, dangerous driving, under eye bags, dehydration, under eye circles, and lower skills leading to errors at work place.

Addictive habits

Avoid certain habits associated with tobacco such as smoking, chewing, snuffing and excess use of alcohol. Substance use disorder is a serious health problem prompting the recommendation to avoid analgesics and opiates, such as oxycodone, hydrocodone, morphine, meperidine and unprescribed drugs such as cocaine, heroin, and synthetic drugs such as fentanyl. A small amount of alcohol consumed in moderation has been acceptable for those who don't have issues with chemical dependency, although even this is a controversial subject.

Studies show that red wine may reduce the risk of heart attacks or atherosclerotic plaque buildup attributed to the chemical resveratrol found in the grape's skin. It is imperative that alcohol not be consumed with sleeping pills, sedatives, or opioid drugs. Binge-drinking is hazardous.

Happiness and peace

According to the Dalai Lama, happiness is a state of mind. Happiness and peace must come from within. Some people will never be happy, no matter how much they own and how much they get. They keep comparing themselves to others. Those who are happy live longer, have less stress, and have fewer diseases.

About half of happiness is an inborn habit. About 10 percent is due to circumstances, and the remaining 40 percent is attributed to one's attitude. This last group can try to make themselves happier by taking the right steps in their outlook. Instead of looking at negatives all the time, they could look at positives. Smiling more often and making small talk with strangers and customers will increase friends. Avoiding controversial topics such as politics or personal matters will reduce tension. Counting one's own blessings in life and recognizing own errors committed in the past will bring peace. Finally accepting destiny or fate or God's will instead of blaming themselves for events that go out of control will reduce mental stress.

Money helps people, up to a certain income level, to feel secure and comfortable, but beyond that, it does not increase happiness. In fact, too much money brings more stress and unhealthy habits and eventual unhappiness. Social activities, volunteerism, enjoying nature, personal accomplishments, and activities are the ways to improve happiness level.

There are four happiness hormones known which can bring about contentment. Endorphin is an activity hormone. Exercise, in any form, allows endorphins to be secreted into blood, making one feel better. Dopamine is an achievement hormone that makes one feel good when a challenging task is accomplished. Serotonin is a socializing hormone that makes one feel better when having friends, social conversations, and group activities. Finally, oxytocin is a touch hormone that makes one feel good even on simple touching.

Five sensations that we know—namely taste, smell, hear, see, and touch—also bring in good feelings. Tasting a good food or drink, smelling good perfume or flower, listening to good music, reading a good book or watching sunset and birds, and hugging and holding hands of a good friend or spouse and holding grandchildren in your laps are all items that bring in happiness, smile, and good feelings. Tapping into these senses is inexpensive or free.

Prayer, meditation

Placing belief on a supreme power, praying to one's chosen God, or following religious rituals and meditating in any fashion are tools available for one to find peace and calm. It may not be for everyone, and others may not believe in these rituals. However, if it works for one, it is best for that person to continue to seek such solace. Irrespective of God or religion, three tenets to follow as per ancient scriptures to live in peace are the following: (1) Cause no harm to others. Such harm could be caused by one's deeds, words or even thoughts. (2) Help someone if you can, and care about others. (3) Accept that the world is chaotic and learn to live in this world the way it is.

Meditation is a form of relaxation of the mind and body. It requires willful effort to control an overactive mind while the thoughts jump through various bits and pieces. It can be practiced anytime anywhere and calms the mind from anxiety and impatience and reduces stress and anger. It helps to lower blood pressure, anxiety, and chronic pain syndromes and thus increases longevity and youthfulness.

Nature

Mother Nature is kind and good to all. It is free for everyone. Sunlight is good for the skin and helps to generate vitamin D. Obviously, one should be careful in avoiding too much sunlight, and use of solar protection, such as sunscreen and hats, is advisable. A Waterfront makes us feel peaceful. We are waterborne animals by evolution; we were in a medium of water in the mother's womb, and our body mass is 80 percent water. No wonder we feel attracted to the beachfront and waterfront. Trees, gardens, flowers, lakes, rivers, mountains, green grass, butterflies and deer, snow, and glaciers; found in nature make us smile and be happy. Being with nature is like being with God and being with Mother. In our daily hurry to make ends meet, we often forget to enjoy what is there and free.

Nature provides good health and longevity. Avoiding pollution will improve health. Longevity is threatened for those who live in polluted areas of the world. Evidence suggests that those who live in highly polluted areas such as New Delhi or Beijing are inhaling bad pollutants equivalent to smoking fifty cigarettes a day. They develop allergic reactions, asthma, and upper respiratory conditions.

Looking good is feeling good

Good grooming, cleanliness, facial hygiene, eyebrows, attire, skin and hair conditioning, and a pleasant smile are all good things, which bring in good company, better social activity, personal self-confidence, and self-esteem. These lead to feeling good, which translates to better mental state and better health. Moisturizing skin cream helps to avoid dryness of skin. Dry skin can lead to itching and scratching, which in turn causes small ulcerations and skin infections. It also causes more skin wrinkling. Properly fitting shoes for walking and for different sporting activities is important to reduce falls and ankle and foot injuries. Showering or bathing regularly reduces surface infections, and proper hair grooming reduces scalp infestations with lice and ticks. Body odor can be repulsive, and it is good to use deodorants.

Independence

Loss of independence is one of the scariest events for an older person. As one loses hearing, vision, cognition, and balance, it becomes necessary to depend on others for daily functions. It becomes quite disheartening, especially when one's mind is still agile. Eight items on the checklist to determine physical independence are: ability to use the toilet, eat, dress, bathe, groom, get out of bed, get out of a chair, and walk. Eight items on the checklist for independent living are the ability to: do shopping, cooking, housekeeping, managing financial matters, doing laundry, making phone calls, traveling, and taking medications. Driving is an added boost. Independence promotes mental comfort and strength.

Hobby

It is desirable to nurture a hobby because it brings in satisfaction, fun, and relaxation. They allow one to interact with others and exercise the body and brain pleasantly. Hobbies encourage one to focus and learn new skills, thus allowing the brain to make new neurons. A hobby should be something one wants and likes to do for fun besides work, thus reducing work-related stress. It can be an exercise or sporting activity. It can also be something creative, like carpentry, architecture, or building. A hobby can be an art such as painting, music, reading, writing, photography, pottery, sculpting, dancing, or acting. It can be volunteering to help others such as at a church or a hospital. It can be games such as bridge, other card games, or chess or board games. Whatever it may be, it is something to enjoy and share with others. If one can share a hobby with your spouse or family member, it adds to your bonding. It will reduce the aging process, allowing one to be socially connected and intellectually engaged.

Dental hygiene

Routine dental care gets limited attention in impoverished countries. Good dental hygiene prevents oral cavity problems and systemic inflammation. Dental flossing is recommended regularly after every meal, and brushing is recommended twice daily. It also improves social interactions and mental confidence. Good dental condition is an indicator of good habits, good hygiene, and good health.

Safety

Prevention of accidents, injuries, and falls is critical. A substantial number of trauma related hospitals admissions are attributed to falls and accidents. The resulting surgical procedures and their untoward consequences are avoidable by being careful. Safe sex and use of condoms can prevent sexually transmitted diseases. Use of seat belts and airbags have reduced injuries sustained in automobile accidents. Wearing head protection such as helmets while riding bicycles or two-wheelers such as scooters and motorcycles or while skiing, rollerblading, or snowboarding is highly recommended. Avoid cell phone use while driving. Texting while driving is illegal in a growing number of states.

Medical checkups and disease management

Control of known chronic medical conditions such as diabetes mellitus, hypertension, respiratory problems, allergic conditions, neurological, or urological problems is preventative health care. It is desirable to have a family doctor who can do routine physical examinations and various tests to ensure good health. Early detection of abnormalities with corrective steps can prevent complications. Lives can be saved, and premature deaths can be avoided. Routine blood tests will detect anemia, chronic blood loss, nutritional deficiencies, blood cancers, diabetes, kidney disease, cholesterol levels and lipids profile, cancers, liver disorders, and certain metabolic disorders. These could go undetected otherwise until an advanced situation arises, which could be life-threatening. Very often, these could be corrected by taking medications or supplements.

There is no age limit to start any wellness measure. Often, people say that they are too old to start these changes. Any time one institutes these wellness measures, diet, exercise, or mental stimulation, benefits will begin to accrue.

Chapter 27

Prevention of Falls

Deaths result from falls. The fall may appear innocuous at first, a minor slip and fall. Older adults break bones or sustain a brain injury resulting in a hospitalization, surgery, and complications that eventually snowball into end of life. Older adults take medications such as anticoagulants or antiplatelet agents, which can lead to greater susceptibility to bleeding. A fall with a fracture or head injury can lead to a hematoma in the soft tissues or in the intracranial space known as a subdural hematoma.

According to a study by Karel Kaplan, a total of 29,688 Americans over age sixty-five died from falls and related problems in 2016. About one in four older adults sustain a serious fall each year, prompting three million visits to emergency departments of hospitals across the country. Once every nineteen minutes, an older adult dies because of injuries sustained during a fall. One reason is demographics. Older adults are living longer, living with multiple medical problems, and are living independently.

In the trauma section of emergency rooms, the number of older adults presenting with falls has surpassed younger people presenting with real trauma. Initially falls at home appear minor but with further evaluation serious problems are uncovered such as fractures, chest injuries, and head injuries. A fall and subsequent interventions can lead to permanent disability or death.

Conditions that make one more likely to fall include the following:

- Older age
- Neurological deficits
- Lower body weakness
- Vitamin D deficiency
- Vision problems
- Hearing problems
- Medication effects
- Alcohol intake
- Drug abuse
- Improper footwear
- Balancing problems
- Attention distractions

- Careless attitude, denial of deficits
- Hypoglycemia, diabetes mellitus
- Osteoporosis making bones brittle and greater risk for fracture
- Arthritis and back pain superimposed on balancing problems

Mobile phones have caused a new set of problems, such as

- listening to music or talking while walking or crossing roads, obscuring warning sounds;
- texting while driving, walking, or climbing into public vehicles;
- playing games such as Pokémon while walking;
- taking pictures and selfies without watching for hazards;
- using headphones or earplugs that reduce sounds of caution; and
- watching videos while walking.

Sporting injuries are another reason for falls. They are higher with contact sports, such as football, basketball, hockey, or soccer. Injuries are higher with skiing, snowboarding, horseback riding, parasailing, bungee jumping, and parachute jumping, where there is less chance of balancing and control by the individual. In addition, one should consider enhanced safety measures in one's home, such as

- living in a one-story house compared to a two-story house with a staircase;
- even flooring throughout the house instead of having steps between rooms;
- area rugs and mats to have flat and tight placements;
- keeping slippers and footwear away from doorsteps and bottom of stairwells;
- installing grab bars in shower stalls, toilets, and other wet areas;
- having handrails on both sides of staircases;
- adequate lighting inside the house;
- keeping the floors with maximum open and walking space instead of cluttering with objects and furniture; and
- keeping the house clean.

Other measures of value are

- balancing exercises and
- having medical checkups to ensure safety.

Fall prevention is practiced in hospitals and nursing homes. It includes proper use of side rails for beds, restraints, sedation, and surveillance cameras. Weight-bearing exercises with strengthening of muscles, balancing exercises, and stretching exercises as in yoga. Evaluation of medications that cause drowsiness, vision problems, and syncope.

Medical conditions such as hypoglycemia in diabetes mellitus, cerebellar problems that affect stability, and Parkinson's disease that cause tremors and ataxia are examples.

CDC has a website for instructions and educational materials at cdc.gov/steadi (which stands for "Stopping elderly accidents, deaths, and injuries"). Another site for information is ncoa.org (National Council on Aging) and enter "falls" in the search box.

Section 5

Compassionate Care of the Older Adult

Venkit S. Iyer, MD and David Bernstein, MD

Chapter 28

Dying with Dignity

Where would you like to die?

When asked, nine out of ten adults would prefer to die in their home, in their familiar surroundings, in their bed, with their family, spouse, and children nearby, and in peace and comfort. There is no doubt this is the best way, but only the fortunate four out of ten achieve it. The rest die in the hospital or nursing home or extended care facilities. The least fortunate ones die in the streets or battlefields or in unknown gutters or similar forsaken places.

Everyone would agree that hospitals are not the desirable place to die with dignity. Too many regulations, too many interruptions, change of personnel, formal attitude, legalities, blood tests, intravenous fluids, tubes and catheters, forceful treatments, inability to sleep due to noise and lights, and nursing care and excessive cost are difficult to endure. Nursing homes and long-term care facilities are for those who do not have families or have families unable to provide them with daily care.

The best place to die with dignity is in one's own home, in bed, cared for by a spouse or other family member. The family may engage a nursing aide to give personal care, such as washing or bathing, but the family member is always there. The blessed ones die in this manner. No one wants to die in the ICU (intensive care unit) of a hospital, but unfortunately one-fifth of Americans die in the hospital ICU, and many more are shuttled through the hospital in the last few months of their lives. (*Surgical Intensive Care Medicine Second Edition*, 2009, by Allan Garland).

However, loved ones are taken to the hospital when they become acutely ill. Family members, health surrogates, and POA want to make sure they are not being neglectful; they want to correct any acute, correctable problems and want to provide emergency care. They hope for compassion. Sad to say, certain medical treatments can be regarded as overly aggressive or even unnecessary for older adults or terminally ill patients. Testing and treatments might be performed either out of fear, ignorance, or greed.

Advances in medicine make it possible to prolong life without meaning or quality. It is up to the family and the family's doctor to avoid hospitalization of a terminally ill individual. This requires planning and getting all concerned on the same page.

There are borderline cases where one can say the life support is excessive but may be justifiable. Timing could be an issue. Should the individual be given another day or another week hoping for recovery? How long to continue antibiotics, how long to continue respiratory support, how long to watch a brain-dead person, how long to continue nutritional support? These are to be decided based on the situation by individual families with advice of treating doctors.

Studies done in the past have shown that many patients endured painful and prolonged deaths due to unjustified heroic life-supporting treatments with no aim or goal (JAMA 1995). Pulling the plug was a taboo and was performed quietly with unspoken words. Aging adults fear is not death itself, but they may die after a prolonged period of agony, pain, and suffering with the inability to communicate with their loved ones in the last few days of their life. They wish to hold them or touch them and want to say goodbye or give last-minute instructions. All these are denied if you are dying in a hospital ICU.

Other situations result in patients being placed into long-term care facilities or adult living facilities. Their family members may be successful, and they may be wealthy but lack the time, interest, or opportunity to care for their older adult parents. Modern societal living has transitioned away from the multigenerational home, where a younger generation provided care to their older family members.

Pain management

Pain presents a significant problem in the aging population. Most aging adults express a desire to die without pain or suffering, but only about half are fortunate to have their pain controlled. It is a humane act to relieve the pain of a terminally ill person. Pain can be because of fractures, nerve compressions, tumor growths, soft tissue infections, musculoskeletal problems, degenerative disorders, or head and neck disorders. For some individuals, pain is constant, and relief may only occur when sleeping. These individuals need adequate pain medications in doses enough to control the pain. Dying with dignity requires an understanding physician and family who will see to it they do not suffer from unnecessary pain. A morphine pump or a PCA (patient-controlled analgesia) would be a valuable adjunct. Morphine is a useful drug for controlling pain for the terminally ill.

Pain management has become a hot topic recently as opioid dependence and abuse has led to over 93,000 deaths a year in the USA in 2020. Twenty years earlier, it was felt that patients were not getting adequate pain control, and Congress approved laws to encourage pain control. Specialties developed purely for pain management with multiple specialties branching off into this field. These physicians perform epidural injections, various nerve blocks, insertion of morphine pumps, and write prescriptions. Pain pill mills evolved just to prescribe oral painkillers such as OxyContin. Later, they added fentanyl and other injectable medications. With the current climate of overprescription, the federal government has limited prescriptions of narcotics as a response to overdoses and deaths due to opiates. Those who are terminally ill and have chronic pain syndromes must be able to get pain medications as needed to keep them comfortable. It is unfair to withhold pain medications from them in the name of avoiding the potential for the development of dependence. Acute pain related to infections, surgery, and trauma must also get adequate pain control in times of need.

Sleep management

Another challenge at the end of life is difficulty with sleeping and agitation. This can be due to neurological or metabolic problems. Anxiety and stress can precipitate depression. Patients nearing the end of life need or benefit from medication for anxiety or sedation. Lack of sleep causes more stress, irritability, and medical and mental problems. Over forty percent of the adult population have insomnia. Fear of suicide and drug dependence leads to inadequate prescriptions for sleep management. During sleep hours, the brain gets much of its required rest. It washes out toxins that accumulate in the brain. This is an opportunity for regeneration and development of new neurons. We all notice how refreshed and energized we feel after a good night's sleep.

After a night of poor sleep, we feel tired, depressed and listless, irritable, and angry. This is well proven by animal experiments, where rats develop illnesses from inadequate sleep. Experts recommend seven to eight hours of sleep each night to support good health.

Empathy

Terminally ill patients are extremely appreciative of words of empathy, kindness, and caring. Friction between patient and caregiver is not uncommon due to the burden of the tasks involved in the process. The last thing terminally ill individuals want to hear is being blamed and feeling neglected due to the burden of providing care. The dying person prefers to die as peacefully as possible.

These patients have neurological disorders, dementia, or Alzheimer's disease. Toxicity of chemicals accumulating in blood from kidney or liver failures can affect the brain function. These patients may be agitated, irrational, forgetful or even violent due to confusion. Instead of restraints, these individuals wish to be treated with kindness, compassion and dignity.

Federal and state regulations require hospitals and nursing homes to avoid restraints, increasing the risk that an agitated or confused patient might fall. Falls from the bed are reportable incidents liable for legal actions against the nurses or hospitals.

There is a difference between prolonging life versus relieving suffering for care of the dying. Dying with dignity means dying in comfort both physically and emotionally. Mere prolongation of life with continued daily suffering from pain, sleeplessness, and discomfort is not worthwhile. This does not mean that one should stop nutrition and fluids or simple medical treatments either. One can die with dignity in the comfort of one's own home without undergoing extraordinary treatment measures, such as dialysis or surgery. It would be necessary to refuse certain types of medical treatments while continuing common sense treatments, particularly pain medications, sedatives, and sleeping aids.

It is important to have someone close and competent designated and authorized to conduct your wishes. Often it may not be an immediate family member who can get emotionally tangled. It could be a nurse or a trusted friend with the help of aides or hired help to provide personal care, bathing, cleaning, bed pans, moving, and so forth. This person might need to take charge of the situation and function as a coordinator, planner, and marshal.

Ultimately, the individual himself or herself also must take moral responsibility for passing with peace and comfort. It is the passage predestined, not to be seen as a struggle and fight for a few more days. With proper planning, with the help of friends and family, and with help from doctors and nurses, one can make it easy for oneself as well as for others. There can be an acceptance with sadness and with a celebration of life.

The entire medical system or health-care field is geared to take care of illnesses, sickness, injuries, accidents, and other acute events. Less emphasis is given to providing well-being, preventative care, and long-term care. Old age and related maintenance issues are not attractive subjects for most physicians. Hospitals expend a huge resource on prolonging the last few days or weeks of life, knowing well in advance that such prolongation of life is only for a fleeting period of time, maybe days or weeks. This care can be regarded as futile. The last three months of a person's life become the most expensive. Even if they survive and go home, they expire in short order. There is an innate refusal to accept the eventuality of death. We consider success as measured by discharge from the hospital alive, not by the quality of life afterward.

Pacemakers and defibrillators (AICD) can be deactivated in a terminally ill patient if that is the only device that is keeping them alive. Experts from American Heart Association and American College of Cardiology have written statements that disabling a pacemaker or defibrillator is neither physician-assisted suicide nor euthanasia. The patient or durable power of attorney has a legal and moral right to request for such deactivation (Lampert, Rachel, et al. HRS expert consensus statement on management of cardiovascular implantable electronic devices in patients nearing the end of life or requesting withdrawal of therapy, Heart Rhythm, July 2010).

For the past twenty to thirty years, there has been a better recognition of palliative care, pain management, hospice care, physiotherapy, and geriatric care. These topics should be taught to all medical students. A limited number of physicians opt for practice in these fields as their chosen specialty. The most crucial element needed here is compassion and kindness and not medicine or surgery. There is also job satisfaction when an impossible and difficult clinical challenge is met with the latest device or technology as compared to just talking to an old adult and making sure he or she is walking, urinating, and having bowel movements. While the doctors can do only so much, the burden is transferred to nurses. The most important people who can do the most, however, are family members.

There is no rule set by nature that all humans must die in a hospital or nursing home. They can die in their homes as they did decades ago.

There is also no rule set by nature that death should be slow and prolonged over a course of days or weeks. If there is adequate time given to family and friends to absorb the news of the impending death, they have adequate time to express sympathy, then this is considered as a good death, a natural death, and an expected one. If the death is sudden, unexpected, then it is considered unnatural and tragic.

There was a time when everyone wanted to die quickly and suddenly so that they could leave this world with minimal suffering and leave without being a burden to the family or society. A quick death was considered as a good death then. Women wanted to die before their husbands so that society would not brand them as widows. However, this attitude has changed.

There was a time when family members cared for older adult individuals in their homes. There was good social interaction between residents in the same village and everyone cared for one another. Everyone knew about one another. Older adults expected dying in their bed with minimal suffering, with little trouble given to their caregivers. These respected citizens felt wanted, respected, and had a word or two of wisdom. There was no need for a death certificate, will, or medical investigation. Everyone accepted it was time for the person to go and conduct a funeral, and the rest of the family moved on.

There are a disproportionate number of individuals dying in the intensive care unit after days and weeks of acute and futile care. It was right to give full-throttle medical care at the onset of their illness. However, after a period of two or three weeks, patients and family lose sight of the big picture and continue to focus on the last few hours or the last day in making the next medical decisions. However, no one knows what and why interventions continue. Family members fall into the conundrum of this activity and feel forced to say yes to all suggestions. They are afraid that they may offend someone otherwise, and they do not want to interfere with physician recommendations. The only person who can see the big picture is the primary care physician or the insurance company who is covering the expenses. Eventually pressure comes down from hospital administration because of financial considerations.

Chapter 29

Living Will, Durable Power of Attorney

A Living Will is a legal document that describes one's own preferences in treatment when faced with end-of-life issues. All individuals, except minor children, are encouraged to have such a document prepared and made known to their immediate family members. The primary care physician should have a copy as well. This will facilitate treatment and health-care management in the desired fashion at the time of need, especially when the patient cannot verbalize the directives or opinions.

The most sought-after directive is whether to continue life-support measures when one is in multiple organ failure and prognosis appears to be bleak. Without such a clear directive, doctors in the hospital or intensive care unit will be compelled to keep the person alive and keep treating the person until natural death occurs. As we know, with advances in medical science, it is possible to provide such life support and keep the person alive for weeks and months.

Such a situation, often when treatment is futile, can cause a tremendous financial burden, and the cost could run into hundreds of thousands of dollars. It is a huge emotional drain on the immediate family, visiting the person in the intensive care unit daily and listening to the nurses and doctors often asking you to sign consents and permits, often explaining in poorly understood medical jargon.

If we believe that death is an unavoidable eventuality and if we believe that dying in dignity at home is better than dying in the intensive care unit with multiple drips and tubes in every orifice, then it is prudent for every person to set up a Living Will. All it says is that when death appears to be imminent and when the medical prognosis is poor and when there is no meaningful hope of having quality of life and when the person cannot make sound decisions because of the illness or health situation, the document made while in a sound state of mind and health is considered a directive. It can clearly state that undue prolongation of life and meaningless life support is not desired.

Such clear directives let the family members and doctors do the right thing without feeling guilty or prejudiced. Otherwise, they may feel that they did not try everything in time of illness to save the person. They may feel legally obligated to continue with their routine work as per hospital protocols for fear of malpractice.

A Living Will clearly defines wishes for individual options for care, what they want, and what they do not want. For example, food and water are routinely administered to everyone even after they have been disconnected from a breathing machine. Hence, it is important to state that you do not wish to prolong life with food and water. This was an issue in several legal cases. Similarly, the individual can select procedures they agree or disagree with. They may not want dialysis but would want a pacemaker inserted.

It is a legal document that the person must execute while in good mental health. In addition, it is best to inform your directives to your next of kin or spouse and your primary care doctor so that when an unexpected situation arises, they can get hold of the Living Will document and have it executed. Any attorney can prepare it as part of other legal documents for estate planning. This information can also be obtained for free on websites or physician offices and used. One does not require an attorney to prepare a Living Will or document advanced directives. Most hospitals have generic forms for Living Will execution. However, it must be in writing; a verbal understanding with the next of kin is not adequate.

There were no Living Wills until 1960. It was a new concept then, and there was vigorous opposition to it from the Catholic church and other right-to-life organizations. It took years for the slow advancement of the concept. Because of rising health-care costs and realization of meaningless prolongation of life and suffering at the end of life, it has now become a very well-accepted standard across the country. Cases of Karen Ann Quinlan and Terri Schiavo (who was in a vegetative state for over fifteen years) and the likes received wide political and media attention.

A Living Will and a proxy or durable power of attorney are recommended for all adults and not just by older adults. One may never know when and where destiny is going to play foul. Accidents and head injuries can happen to anyone.

It is the responsibility of patients or families to inform the hospital and treating doctors about the existence of a Living Will. As a corollary, it is the responsibility of the hospital or doctor to ask the patient if they have a Living Will and document that in the admission records. It may sound silly for minor illnesses. But one will never know when a catastrophe will occur. But it is incredibly important for those who have terminal illnesses or advanced age.

A particular scenario is when the doctors write "Do not resuscitate" or DNR order in the chart. This alerts all nurses and other health-care professionals that no CPR (cardiopulmonary resuscitation) is to be performed on the patient if the heart stops. Without such an order, they will call a code when all team members rush in, do chest compressions, give electrical shock, give medications, and insert a tube in the breathing passage to put on a ventilator and so forth. Afterward, the patient is kept on life support until a more definite decision is made.

A dilemma occurs when a person who is on DNR order must go for a procedure in the operating room. Some anesthesiologists insist on having the DNR order rescinded for the duration of surgery and then reinstated at once afterward. This is out of fear of malpractice and legal issues for doing something or not doing something in the operating room. Their argument is that surgery and anesthesia are by itself an invasion with resuscitation, and sometimes a cardiac arrest can happen even for a healthy person because of medication or ventilation issues. Still, there is no justification for doing CPR (cardiopulmonary resuscitation) in the operating room on a patient with prior DNR orders and a Living Will. A frank discussion with patient and family, empathy, and a realistic approach is needed instead of changing paperwork. These patients need intervention despite their illness or advanced age for pain control or palliation or management of injuries. The patients and families very well understand and know that they are in a terminal state, and death is imminent. They are just looking for less suffering and an improved quality of life in the last days.

There are several ways to set up a Living Will. Advance directive forms are available on websites of all state governments for free. Another site is MyDirectives.com, which has a cloud-based digital directive service to cover Living Will, health-care proxy, and organ donation, which are legal in all states. All physician offices, hospitals, and surgery centers have a copy that one can sign on admission. All attorneys have formal documents for execution. One can also compose handwritten directives the same as wills.

Durable power of attorney

This is a legal document that is prepared as a companion to the earlier document of Living Will. In this document, one appoints a certain individual or agent to function as the person's surrogate if and when a situation arises that renders the person unable to decide on his or her own health care.

For example, one sustains a head injury in an automobile accident, requiring emergency surgery, and is in a comatose state for days or weeks. The person named as the durable power of attorney can sign all the consents and permits, which are required by the hospitals. If there was no such document, they usually go by the order of next-of-kin protocol. First in line would be a spouse, then children of bloodline, then siblings. If there were no one available, then they would look for a legal guardian. If none were noted, then they would ask the risk management department to get a court-appointed legal guardian.

Sometimes we have experienced situations where the spouse is divorced or disinterested or demented. Children may be in distant cities. It is good to have someone you trust and dependable to take care of your affairs.

It is important once again to have the document prepared by an attorney and have your desires communicated with the named person. This can avoid unforeseen circumstances and emergencies during care and end-of-life issues.

Like a Living Will, this document was a new concept in the 1980s. California passed the first law allowing durable power of attorney in 1983, and they named it as the Medical Proxy Law. It makes sense since any individual may become unable to express his or her wishes. The Medical Proxy is accepted as a valid legal document in all the states in the country.

Chapter 30
Palliative Care

Palliative care is a multidisciplinary approach to help individuals with life-limiting conditions with the goal of improving quality of life rather than prolonging life. It focuses on relieving pain, physical and mental strain, using the help of doctors, nurses, therapists, and other paramedical personnel.

The word *palliation* or *palliative care* is often used to describe the purpose of a certain type of treatment or surgery to describe that it is being done for symptom relief or for improving the success of other adjuvant therapies but with no expectation of cure. For example, surgeons undertake procedures for palliation when a cure is not expected for cancer patients. Such surgical procedures include debulking (removing chunks of cancer but not all of it) a tumor for better effectiveness of chemotherapy, doing bypass procedures without removing the tumor to overcome blockage of the lumen by the tumor, placing feeding tubes to maintain nutrition, or inserting a morphine pump for continuous infusion of pain medications.

During palliative treatment, medications are provided for vomiting, dizziness, diarrhea, insomnia, and for pain to ease symptoms. Besides cancers, palliative care is provided for treating chronic debilitating conditions such as chronic pulmonary disease, chronic heart disease, degenerative arthritis, and neurological problems, or HIV/AIDS. Palliative care is an approved subspecialty of internal medicine with board certification for those interested in the field.

Palliative care differs from long-term care, end-of-life care, and hospice care even though there may be overlap between them. Palliative care does not automatically mean death is imminent. It can be provided in the hospital, nursing home, or at home. It is a planned and coordinated approach to make the patient more comfortable knowing well that the underlying health problem is not curable, and the patient may live an undetermined length of time.

Symptom assessment is described in Edmonton Symptoms Assessment Scale (ESAS). The symptoms assessed are pain, vomiting or nausea, depression, anxiety, appetite, sense of well-being, activity, drowsiness, and shortness of breath. Palliative care can be provided to children and the pediatric population in addition to adults.

Those in the public confuse alternative medicine or complementary medicine with palliative medicine. Such practices fall outside of the conventional modern medical advice unproven by scientific evidence. However, these practices are widely followed by a vast number of people, either out of blind faith or because of the ineffectiveness of modern medicine or they offer cheap and informal treatment. The so-called placebo effect is a well-known entity. Over time, these techniques have received wider acceptance and are being integrated into modern medical practices.

Chapter 31

Long-Term Care

Long-term care involves a variety of services designed to meet a person's health or personal care needs during a short or prolonged period. These services help people live as independently and safely as possible when they can no longer perform everyday activities on their own. The individual may need help with eating, bathing, ambulating, medication, physiotherapy, and nursing care. Such care can range from home health service to adult day care, adult living facilities, and nursing homes.

When one reaches a certain age with diminished ability to remain independent or when a person sustains an injury or suffers from a life-threatening illness leaving the person debilitated or when one needs help because of dementia or Alzheimer's disease, it becomes necessary to consider options for long-term care.

There are graded levels of care available. A joint decision between the individual and family members, along with the primary doctor, can sort out the options. Other considerations include the financial and insurance status of the individual regarding what services are covered or what is affordable.

Options to consider are home health aides and nursing care, adult living facilities, nursing home care, and hospice care. The choices depend on the level of help needed, such as balance and walking, cognitive status, disabilities, medical conditions, availability of own family members, life expectancy, and financial status.

The simplest level is to get housekeeping help where an assistant or housekeeper can come in to clean the house, cook meals, and do errands. Home health nursing care is useful for someone taking multiple medications, to check on medical state, wound care, or blood pressure. Getting help at home is the least expensive choice. Another possibility is to move in with one of their children and set boundaries about privacy and independence while still needing help with activities of daily living.

There are various low-cost ways of getting help at home. The Retired Senior Volunteer program is a federally funded program to help less mobile senior citizens. "Meals on Wheels" delivers hot nutritious food once a day for a small fee. Website services and online food chains are now available providing fully cooked or partially cooked food and groceries delivered to the door. Online retailers like Amazon can reduce the need to go to department stores and supermarkets for ordinary supplies. Senior citizen centers are helpful sources of information, activities, and food.

Adult day-care centers can be a good supplement to home care. They provide daytime monitoring, meals, personal care, exercises, social companionship, and adult recreation activities. They can be half day or full day and can be one to five days a week. This will help the working children to get time off for them without worrying about their parents. One could call 877-745-1440 or check online, *www.nadsa.org*, for National Adult Day Services Association Inc. Senior centers in one's neighborhood are excellent resources. They provide social and recreational activities, education, and information. Meals may be available as well.

Independent living facilities are usually restricted to seniors living on common grounds who have independent kitchens for limited cooking in the apartments with meal services available on premises and a variety of other assistive services. One step further is assisted living where care is provided to the resident, usually complete cooking, housekeeping, and medical care, but each person is independent. Hospice care is for those having only six months or less to live.

Skilled nursing homes are for those who are totally disabled and require round-the-clock personal care, nutritional support, and medical care, including physical therapy. Some skilled nursing facilities are affiliated with hospitals in different forms. They can be a subacute care facility or step-down unit, or the facility can provide skilled nursing care inside the hospital but with separate admission records. A nursing home can also be a freestanding building, independent of a hospital. One should evaluate the reputation of the facility and make a personal site visit before selecting a facility.

Long-term care insurance policies are promoted and advertised as a backup resource when the need arises. There are pros and cons to consider before one buys a policy. It is up to each individual to make an informed decision on this after consulting his or her financial planners and family. In general, these policies are profitable for insurance companies if one calculates the total premium paid and the total payout. It is a way of having peace of mind and a sense of security, but many will never use it or use only a portion of it. They are often not financially good investments and can be expensive to start with. One is recommended to read all the provisions, exemptions, riders, and conditions carefully before signing on to one.

Medicare and Medicaid cover portions of long-term care. Following a hospitalization for major illness or surgery, short-term home health, physiotherapy, or skilled nursing home admission are covered. Usually, these services are fully covered for the first twenty days and partially for the next one hundred days. Hospice care is fully covered for six months. Medicaid rules vary from state to state, and coverage is tied to the income level of the individual.

To get help in deciding and in choosing the most suitable choice for one's needs, a discussion with the individual's primary care physician and family members is advisable. Word of mouth referrals from friends or acquaintances are helpful. Clergy, church, senior centers, and county family agencies are other sources of information. Agency on Aging is a government-funded program. One could call 800-677-1116 or look online at *www.eldercare.gov*. One must take into consideration specific medical needs, cognitive state, personal care needs, and financial obligations in choosing the type of program.

Caregiving can be a difficult and expensive task. Because of the cost and the emotional levels, caregiving often falls on the shoulders of family members. It can lead to stress and interference with their own life and family and affect their health. It is estimated that sixteen million unpaid and undocumented caregivers are taking care of someone in America. There is a need to find positive ways to reduce the stress of caregiving by talking about it with friends.

Chapter 32
Hospice Care

Hospice is a federal-government-supported health and comfort care program for those who are terminally ill and have less than six months to live. Medicare picks up the tab irrespective of previous insurance status. President Reagan signed the Medicare hospice bill in 1981. Since then, there have been no changes to it.

Hospice is derived from Latin *hospes*, meaning guests and hosts, and was known from the Middle Ages when pilgrims were comforted during their journey on religious trips from which they often never returned home. The modern-day hospice was first started in London in 1967. The first American hospice care was started in 1974 in New Haven, Connecticut. Today, the word hospice stands for the philosophy or principles of end-of-life comfort measures rather than structures or buildings.

The National Hospice Organization describes hospice as a holistic, collaborative program of care, which seeks to treat and comfort terminally ill patients and their families at home or in homelike settings. The theme of hospice is comfort care with emotional and spiritual support.

To qualify for the hospice care, the primary care doctor must certify that the person is terminally ill with less than six months to live and refer the patient to a hospice program. The patient must agree for comfort measures only with no further active therapy for the illness. Once it is established that the patient has exhausted all meaningful treatments and that there is no point in continuing maximum efforts to prolong life, it makes sense for the patients to seek pain-free comfort care in the last few weeks or months of their life and to die in peace and with dignity in their home. An example of such a situation will be someone who has advanced cancer, which has spread all over the body and has already been treated with surgery, chemotherapy, and other modalities, to no avail. In 2010, about 1.58 million people in the USA received hospice care services.

Often patients and family members have a wrong impression that by accepting hospice you have given up all hope, all treatments, and you are now embracing death. This is not true. Under hospice, one can continue to receive pain medications, nutrition, various comfort measures, and certain acute therapies. A difference of opinion between a patient, the hospice doctor, and the patient's own primary care physician can arise. Often it is from miscommunication and misunderstandings. If a hospice patient falls and sustains a fracture or gets an acute infection, certainly they are admitted to the hospital and treated. They may even undergo surgery to provide palliation and reduce pain and suffering. But the hospice may not agree to intensive chemotherapy. Hospice provides reasonable care for palliation and management of terminal illness and related conditions.

Before entering hospice care, one should make sure all curable options have been considered in managing any illness. One should never give up hope and get second opinions, when necessary, especially if the first opinion is disheartening. There can be mistakes or misinformation. The test results need to be verified for accuracy and reliability. What is treatable at one hospital or medical center may be regarded as untreatable at another center and vice versa. One should review the pathology slides and make sure the diagnosis is confirmed as cancer. For a first-time diagnosis of cancer, one may choose an aggressive approach with radical surgery, radiation, chemotherapy, or other newer modalities. One should explore all avenues, do the maximum, and follow it up with necessary tests and recommendations.

When considering hospice with advanced, end-stage cancer and all options have been exhausted, it becomes time to be more realistic about survival. It is at this stage that a consensus between all family members and doctors has been accepted. It is now time to talk about palliative care and comfort measures to avoid more pain and suffering and look toward peace, and a higher power.

Five Cs for hospice care are communication, collaboration, compassionate care, comfort, and cultural care (spirituality).

Most common location of the hospice care is the patient's own residence. It can also be in a hospice in-patient facility or assisted living facility or nursing home or in the hospital itself in designated areas. According to a report presented by the National Hospice and Palliative Care Organization in 2012, 66.4 percent received their care in their residence and 26.1 percent in a hospice facility. An approved hospice program that is chosen by the patient takes over the entire care, which provides a physician, nurse, and other health-care workers as needed. Hospice provides medications, medical equipment, hospital bed, nutritional support, and other personal care services. Hospice will also provide physiotherapy, speech therapy, and emotional support as needed. They will not do housekeeping or cooking.

They will continue to provide medical care for other coexisting medical conditions, provide pain medications, and monitor vital signs. The nurses provide care with input from the hospice physician and the primary care physician if needed. It is possible to switch from one hospice program to another one if there is disagreement or dissatisfaction with the first one. The hospice organization might be able to help with funeral plans and arrangements.

Once a hospice team has accepted the patient, they take over the entire care in consultation with the primary doctor or other treating doctors and family members. A team of health-care experts arrives, which includes a hospice doctor, nurse, social worker, counselor, chaplain, home health aid, and trained volunteers.

The US Congress enacted the Medicare hospice benefit in 1986 and in 1993. They established it as a component of all health-care government provisions. Medicare covers almost all of hospice care. There is a small copay often. Medicaid and most private health insurances also cover hospice. Medicare advantage programs can turn over the care to regular Medicare while under hospice. The regular insurance will continue to cover unrelated medical problems. In fact, it is wiser to keep paying the premiums to Medicare A and B and to keep the Medicare advantage plan or other private insurances active in case the hospice ends. It may be difficult to re-enroll at the time of dire need afterward. For example, one may be under hospice care for terminal cancer. But if there is a broken bone from a fall, that will be fixed under Medicare or regular insurance. One can voluntarily decide to relinquish hospice and return to regular care at any time. Sometimes the person may live more than six months and disenroll from hospice and later re-enroll when the situation worsens.

Hospice care and end-of-life palliative care have helped to reduce medical expenses significantly. About 30 percent of Medicare expenses are spent in the last year of an individual's life. ER visits and hospitalizations are avoided along with limited value tests and treatments. A proposal was made to cover end-of-life consultations as a reimbursable fee-for-service to physicians under the Affordable Care Act, and it is now a reimbursable charge.

We have heard of famous people who made common sense decisions to die at home with friends and family in their own bed and with comfort.

Senator John McCain was diagnosed with brain cancer, a glioblastoma. He underwent tests and initial treatments. On August 24 of 2018, he stopped all treatment for the cancer and entered hospice care. His decision was lauded as a wise decision since the cancer was incurable, steadily growing, and with imminent death.

Jackie Kennedy and Barbara Bush died within two days of the announced withdrawal of further medical treatments. Both their homes were open for visitors, friends and family. Both had a dignified funeral with state and national honor. The publicity they received following such dignified death should give confidence to the average citizens to accept hospice care as a comforting choice. Hospice care is different from giving up hope or hastening death. It is accepting realities and doing the best under the circumstances.

Hospice care addresses physical, emotional, medical, social, and spiritual needs for those facing life-limiting illnesses. They also provide counseling to family members and caregivers on issues such as cleaning the house and shopping. Hospice does not limit medical care, but it focuses on quality of life instead on trying to cure the incurable. A chaplain or religious priest may visit the person.

How to find the hospice that works for you? The easiest way is to ask your doctor or nurses or ask your friends who had used them in the past. One can go through Internet web searches. One can also call 1-800-658-8898 for the National Hospice and Palliative Care Organization. For languages other than English, the phone number is 1-877-658-8896. Once you select an organization, make sure you ask questions to your satisfaction before you sign up with them. Specifically, you want to know round-the-clock availability of health-care workers in times of need and emergency and their history in the community you live in.

Chapter 33

Prevention of Infections and Infestations

Simple and inexpensive preventive measures and precautions can reduce infections and infestations. Millions of people die or become disabled from infections and infestations every year. Simple common-sense measures can prevent this calamity. Community education and uplifting impoverished people from unhealthy and unsanitary surroundings will save thousands of lives.

Food

Many of the infestations are through contaminated food. Roundworms, pinworms, Shigella dysentery, salmonella and typhoid, cholera, amebiasis, and food poisoning are through unclean, unhealthy, or contaminated food. Mechanically washing the food thoroughly or boiling the food will resolve much of this.

Water

Portions of the world population rely on water from tanks, wells, and rivers since they have no other sources of water. Very often these water sources are contaminated, carrying deadly bacteria. Cholera and schistosomiasis are examples. The water requires filtration and boiling before consumption.

Sanitation

In rural areas without toilet facilities residents relieve themselves in open fields. This leads to contamination of ground water, agricultural products, and food items. In addition, this practice also leads to the infection of secondary hosts such as dogs and pigs, which then transmits infections back to humans. Community education and clean sanitation facilities will alleviate this issue.

Footwear

Walking on bare feet outdoors can lead to the penetration of the skin on the soles by Helminthes, leading to hookworm infections. They also lead to injuries, secondary bacterial infection, and abscess formation.

Handwashing

Simple handwashing with soap and water kills viruses and cleanses the hands from bacteria, dirt, and parasites. Handwashing is particularly important before eating food and after touching any contaminated surfaces. Food handlers and cooks in restaurants are to be extra careful in frequent handwashing.

Safe sex

Wearing a condom will markedly reduce sexually transmitted diseases such as HIV/AIDS, pelvic inflammatory disease, syphilis, and gonorrhea. Condoms will also reduce unwanted pregnancies.

Body wash

Cleansing the body twice a day helps clear off all surface contaminations, sweat, and smell. It reduces the chances for lice and ticks, which cause skin infections.

Mosquito nets

Mosquito and insect borne infections are prevalent throughout the world. They include malaria, filariasis, dengue, and chikungunya. Avoiding mosquito bites reduces the chances of contracting such infections.

Insect repellents

A variety of bites and stings by bugs and insects transmit infections and cause abscess formation. Houseflies can contaminate food. Tsetse flies spread leishmaniasis.

Gloves

Working in the garden, woods, and soil is better done while wearing gloves. This reduces nail-bed contamination, which can cause infections. Gloves are also useful in health care to prevent cross contamination.

Masks

Wearing masks helps prevent the transmission of airborne infections such as influenza, COVID-19, Spanish flu, and chicken flu. Droplets while coughing, sneezing, or laughing make the transmission happen.

Laundry

Washing clothes with bleach and water and then hot ironing them afterward will reduce the transmission of infections from soiled clothes. Clothes worn by an infected person will have the organisms clinging to them from body secretions, stool, urine, and blood.

Vaccination

Vaccines are easily available to prevent diseases such as smallpox, measles, diphtheria, tetanus, poliomyelitis, COVID-19, influenza, yellow fever, and shingles. DPT was for diphtheria, pertussis (whooping cough) and tetanus; MMR was for measles, mumps, and rubella.

Isolation and quarantine

Keeping your distance from an infected person helps prevent further spread and helps contain the infection in the community.

Cleanliness

Keeping the house clean and tidy reduces the chance of encountering pests such as roaches (among other insects and bugs), lizards, snakes, and rats in your environment.

Fumigations and insecticides

Measures to kill bugs and insects using insecticides and other chemicals will reduce bedbugs, ticks, mosquitoes, and other creatures.

Garbage disposal

Proper garbage disposal prevents the growth and inhabitance of larvae, mosquitoes, flies, rodents, and reptiles, which can cause injuries to humans.

Control of stray animals

Stray dogs, monkeys, and other animals can cause bites and injuries, transmitting infections.

Safety precautions

Avoid going into the wilderness alone. Feeding alligators and other wild animals, walking without footwear in shallow waters, touching unknown plants and shrubs, and petting undomesticated animals are all invitations for injuries, bites, and infections.

Avoid body contact

Contagious diseases can be contracted from touching an infected person. Sometimes it is due to sexual contact; sometimes it is due to sharing needles, beds, or clothing. Very often it is from shaking hands or hugging strangers.

Avoid unnecessary travels

Travel causes contact with others, hours of stay in close and crowed quarters or vehicles, and disruptions in daily routines and hygienic measures.

Avoid unnecessary crowds

Crowded places increase body contact, injuries, and stress. Whenever possible, plan to avoid crowds.

ABOUT THE AUTHORS

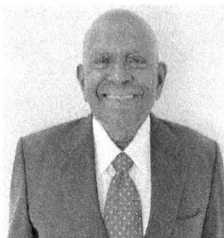

Venkit S. Iyer MBBS, MS Surgery, FACS, FRCS-C, FICS

Venkit S. Iyer MBBS, MS Surgery, FACS, FRCS-C, FICS is a highly respected physician born in Palakkad District, Kerala State, in India. His parents emphasized the value of education. This enabled him to achieve a higher education and admission to medical college. After completing his medical degree in 1967, he went on to complete post-graduation (master's degree) in surgery. He later migrated to the United States for higher education and training in surgery.

He completed an internship and residency in New York and started working at the same hospital as a full-time teaching faculty member in the department of surgery. After a year of work and teaching at Albert Einstein College of Medicine, Bronx, New York, he moved to Florida, starting a consulting private practice in general and vascular surgery. For thirty years, he practiced surgery in Palm Harbor, Florida, retiring in 2014. Since then, he has participated in various medical missions and other charitable work.

Dr. Iyer is the author of the following books:

- **Decision Making in Clinical Surgery:** This practical guide helps medical students, interns, and residents navigate surgical challenges.
- **Aging Well and Reaching Beyond:** This accessible book empowers the public to make informed decisions about their health and well-being.
- **The Clinic:** This thought-provoking exploration delves into complex medical issues through a fictional narrative.

- **Geriatrics Handbook** (co-authored): A resource for understanding and caring for older adults.
- **Iyer's Storybook for Children Vol. 1 and Vol. 2:** Engaging illustrations and healthcare messages make learning fun for young readers.

Dr. Iyer's dedication to his profession and his commitment to sharing knowledge are evident from his accomplishments.

Dr. Venkit S. Iyer is a board-certified surgeon, Fellow of American College of Surgeons (FACS), Fellow of Royal College of Physicians and Surgeons of Canada (FRCS-C), and Fellow of International College of Surgeons (FICS). He has held leadership positions, teaching positions, and lectures and educates in various forums. Dr. Iyer has also authored articles in various journals and magazines.

Dr. Iyer lives in Palm Harbor, Florida.
He can be contacted via email at venkitiyer@gmail.com.
Website venkitiyer.com

*****

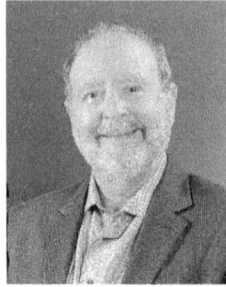

David Bernstein, MD FACP

David Bernstein MD is a highly respected, award-winning physician and author who is board certified in both internal medicine and geriatrics practicing in Clearwater, Florida. His forty plus years of experience have provided him with opportunities to observe and empathize with thousands of adults as they age. His insight and ability to monitor patient patterns and outcomes compelled him to share what he has learned with others.

Dr. Bernstein is a graduate of Albany Medical College. He has served as chairperson of his hospital's Pharmacy and Therapeutic Committee for twenty years, helping to improve patient safety and outcomes. As an associate clinical professor in the department of medicine at the University of South Florida College of Medicine, he has taught the skills he has acquired over the years to first and second-year students.

His publications include the following:

- **I've Got Some Good News and Some Bad News: You're OLD, Tales of a Geriatrician, What to Expect in Your 60s, 70s, 80s, and Beyond** shares his acronym GRACE to describe the five secrets for leading a happier, healthier, longer life so we can all *age gracefully*®. "A necessary, straightforward read for all ages, since life, as Bernstein bluntly states, is a process of coming-of-old-age" *(Kirkus Reviews)*.
- **Senior Driving Dilemmas, Lifesaving Strategies** is an informational guide to families, helping them understand the complexities of senior driving.

- **The Power of 5: The Ultimate Formula for Longevity and Remaining Youthful.** Dr. Bernstein uses five words that begin with the letter *S* to describe the ultimate formula he knows can save your life.
- **The Power of 5: A Journal for a Journal for Health, Longevity and Wellness,** providing a guide to integrating The Power of 5 formula into one's life.
- **Geriatrics Handbook (co-authored):** A resource for understanding and caring for older adults.

Dr. Bernstein is an engaging and entertaining public speaker. He addresses various medical topics with his colleagues and with the community at large with a focus on individuals and families facing the complex problems of aging and staying healthy and youthful.

David Bernstein MD lives in Tampa, Florida, with his wife, Melissa. He can be contacted via email at david@powerof5life.com

Social Media:
Website: PowerOf5Life.com
Facebook: Facebook.com/PowerOf5Life
LinkedIn: www.LinkedIn.com/inDavidbernstein2200/
Twitter: www.Twitter.com/DBernsteinMD
Instagram: www.Instagram.com/drdavidbernstein
YouTube: https://www.youtube.com/@powerof5life453/video
Substack: BernsteinsPowerof5Life.Substack.com

www.ingramcontent.com/pod-product-compliance
Lightning Source LLC
Chambersburg PA
CBHW031121020426
42333CB00012B/176